Why We Get Sick

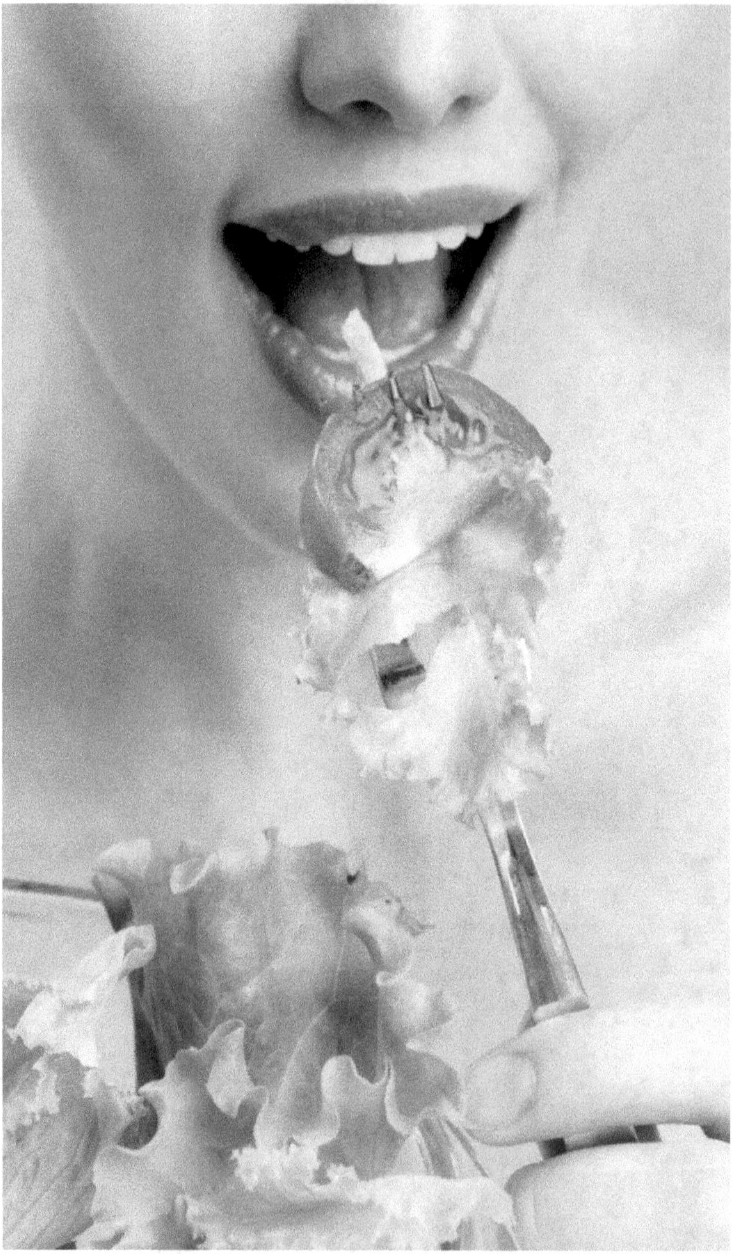

Why We Get Sick

Principles that Will Change Your Diet and Improve Your Health

Rossie C Pattison

Copyright Notice

This book is a general educational health-related information product. As an express condition to reading this book, you understand and agree to the following terms. The books content is not a substitute for direct, personal, professional medical care and diagnosis.

Please see your doctor or health care provider if you are unsure of eating any of the foods in this book or participating in any of the activities as everyone has different health care needs and concerns.

The Author and/ or Publisher of this book is not responsible in any manner whatsoever for any consequential damages that result from the use of, or the inability to use this book.

First Printing, 2014

ISBN-13: 978-1497538252

Contents

Preface: The Foundation of Good Nutrition

The human anatomy is a complicated organism which has the capability to heal itself-if you take the time to listen to it and react with proper nourishment and care. Despite most of the mistreatment our bodies suffer-whether through exposure to toxins, or inactivity-they still often serves us well for a long time before hints of sickness may begin to appear. Even then, using a tiny bit of help, they respond and keep functioning.

Good nutrition is the basis of healthiness. Everyone should have these four fundamental nutrients in their daily diet-proteins, carbohydrates, fats, water-and also vitamins, minerals, along with other micronutrients. You have to possess a good notion of the mixtures of a wholesome diet, to help you to better comprehend why those foods must be supported with nutritional supplement, and to select the appropriate foods.

It's no necessity in the USA that all package foods of nutrition label that tells the customer what's truly inside the package. This system might not be ideal, but it's a huge advancement over no tagging at all.

Remember, that all clean, minimally-processed foods, for example grains bought in volume, meats, fruits, and veggies, usually do not take labels. Since they've more valuable nutrients and fewer unsafe ones, nevertheless they are naturally healthier in comparison to package meals.

Think of the body as being made up of numerous tiny small machines. Many of these machines function in harmony; some operate alone. For the machine to function correctly, they demand fuels. The machine won't execute to its optimal ability, when the kind of fuel giving is the erroneous combination.

Our body's fuel comes from the things we eat on a daily basis. If the machine is offered no fuel, it'll eventually stop working. Foods consist of many nutrients and it is important to consume as much nutrients as possible.

We can get these nutrients from water, minerals, enzymes, lipids, vitamins, carbohydrates, and proteins. It's these nutriment's that sustain our body by giving us the essential materials the body need to carry on with everyday functions.

Based On scientific researcher, bone is one of the strongest building materials known to man. If your leg muscles move as rapidly as your eye muscles, you could walk more than 50 miles in one day.

Recent studies have demonstrated that each part of the human's body contains very high concentrations of specific nutriments. Although nutriment's has various special purposes, their main purpose is really to keep us going.

A lack of those nutriments will cause the body part to breakdown and eventually start to malfunction-and, subsequently other parts of the body will follow soon after.

Individual nutritional elements vary in form and function, as well as in the amount needed by the human body; nevertheless, they are all essential to our health.

The activities that demand nutriment's take place on microscope levels, and the specific procedures vary considerably. Nutriments are involved in all-body processes, from restoring tissue to thinking and combating disease.

To keep this from occurring, we are need the correct diet and right nutritional supplements. With assistance from a well-balanced diet, workout, and also the appropriate nutrients, we could slow the aging procedure and significantly enhance our opportunities to get a healthier, pain-free-and longer-life.

If we do not give the body the appropriate nutriments, we could impair the body's regular functions and bring great harm to ourselves. We might not always be healthy, even when we have no signs of sickness. May be that we're not yet showing any obvious symptoms of sickness.

One trouble most people have is that we don't get the nutriments we need from our diet plans because all of the foods we eat are processed. Cooking foods at high temperatures ruins the essential nutriments the body needs to work correctly. The all-natural, uncooked foods that provide these components are mostly missing from the diet.

The past years as revealed, much new understanding concerning nutrition and its impacts on the human's body, as well as the role it plays in illness. Phytochemicals are substances present in plants that make the plans biologically active. Or vegetables and fruits consist of phytochemicals.

Yet, as few individuals eat sufficient fruits and vegetables to obtain the optimum quantity of phytochemicals from diet alone, supplementation is recommended. Phytochemicals or not nutriments in the traditional sense, but they establish a plants color, taste, and ability to withstand disease.

Analysts have established the technology to draw out these chemical compounds and concentrate them into tablets, powders, and pills.

These products are featured under the term "nutraceuticals." Your body's nutritional requirements are as special to you as your appearance is. The very first essential action to wellness is to make sure you're obtaining the correct amounts of the appropriate nutriments. By knowing the concepts of alternative nourishment and recognizing exactly what nutriments you need, you can boost the state of your wellness and ward off disease.

Introduction

Food Essentials, Our Greatest Medicine

You can't ignore the nature that made your body, knowing what would safeguard it against disease and suffering. Not long ago one of the better known women's magazines, which enjoy a large circulation, published an article exposing the scourge of "unnecessary operations."

The statements and revelations made in this article were strong, far stronger than I have been permitted to make publicly in my years of crusading against the needless use of drugs and surgery, when nutritional therapy could bring far better, safer results with no suffering, and at a price the average man's pocketbook could afford.

Yet neither the author of this article denouncing "unnecessary operations" nor the magazine in which it appeared has been sued for making "false and libelous statements," an action which certainly would have followed any inaccuracy in the accumulation of data.

In fact, many leading members of the medical profession endorsed and corroborated even the strongest statements made by the author. They agreed that of the nine million surgical operations performed every year in America, far too many are not only unnecessary, but "unethically" recommended.

Faulty diagnosis, a wish to experiment surgically, or an inexcusable greed for surgical fees has caused thousands upon thousands of Americans to submit to surgical butchery. It may come as a shock to you to learn that the United States has the highest death rate following surgery of any civilized country.

Too many of our "surgeons" are better businessmen than they are humanitarians and healers. Surgery has become "big business."

In one hospital alone, it was revealed through pathological examination of the removed parts that 28 out of 35 sacrificed appendices were perfectly normal.

The author of the article in question makes the unequivocal statement that "vain and neurotic patients, sloppy diagnosticians and mercenary surgeons have combined to make appendectomy the biggest surgical racket of all time."

In this connection, I take personal and professional pleasure in quoting from an earlier book of mine a statement which, at the time, occasioned much caustic indignation among some of the medical profession, although some months later the same statement, in even stronger form, was to receive the endorsement of many ethical physicians:

No doubt you have read or been told through supposedly authentic sources that the appendix is a "biological mistake"; that it serves no purpose in the body, and really should be removed. Even men who know better are often guilty of making these remarks about the human appendix.

To say that the appendix is a mistake in the human system is to imply that the Creator was asleep on the job and slipped up in this one instance.

I, for one, find it hard to believe that the all-powerful, all-knowing Creator who designed our bodies threw in the appendix for no reason at all. [Incidentally, the same thing holds true for the tonsils, which have been so much maligned by "specialists" during the past decade or two.]

There is good and sufficient reason for every part, both large and small, of the entire human body.

Many persons, who have gotten rid of their "biological mistake" by having their appendix removed, have realized later that they never felt quite the same again!

Their general health has certainly not been improved merely by divorcing themselves from their appendix. Many of them begin to experience chronic constipation and other gastro-intestinal difficulties.

Hundreds of operations on sinuses, stomachs, gall bladders, spleens, intestines, thyroid glands and even on brains are performed every year to relieve symptoms caused by nothing more serious than allergies or nervous and mental upsets.

With too many physicians, the first recourse is to surgery nature and common sense run a losing race. Yet I find a hopeful sign in the fact that a family magazine published by the American Medical Association is containing more and more articles on nutritional therapy, the type of healing in which I have pioneered for years on lecture platforms and through my written words.

For the first time, many American homes will become acquainted, through the medium of this magazine, with articles on preventing and healing bodily ills by means of food elements.

Chapter 1

Nutritional Therapy

Nutritional therapy, at long last, may attain the widespread recognition that it merits, now that many members of the medical profession are ready to acknowledge the inadequacy of drug and surgical therapy as exclusive healing methods.

Thus the outlook for America's health becomes brighter than it has since the day when drugs and surgery usurped the rightful place held by food and herbs as nature's own medicines.

Obviously, there are occasions when surgery or the use of drugs is necessary, and the same holds true with the methods practiced by psychiatry. But the doctors and the psychiatrists must learn that they cannot bypass nutritional therapy entirely, if they hope to achieve a maximum of success with their patients.

Food is nature's own instrument for maintaining and repairing health in human bodies. Our systems were constructed to respond, not to drugs or to the surgeon's knife, but to the vital elements of food.

It was protein, minerals and other nutritive elements contained in food that kept us a living, breathing fetus in our mother's womb and it is these same vitally needed food elements that should keep us healthy and vigorous throughout childhood, the adult years and old age.

All too often our medical practitioners rely upon drugs when a little more thought and open-mindedness would convince them that the only hope for a patient's recovery depended upon nutritional therapy.

For instance, the drug belladonna will "quiet" an irritable bowel; but only the healing influence of certain food elements will remove that bowel's so-called "irritability." Aspirin will relieve temporarily a "nervous" headache, but aspirin will not feed and soothe starved nerve cells.

Benzedrine will "take away" an abnormal desire for food in obese persons, but Benzedrine will not furnish the protein that alone can satisfy the cravings of hidden hunger.

There is much that each person can do to safeguard his or her own health. Obviously, I cannot "prescribe" for anyone, nor are the succeeding paragraphs written with this thought in mind.

Instead, I cite them solely as reminders and to acquaint you with the wonderful work that is being done with natural food elements as remedies and preventives for many human ills.

Your own personal physician may or may not agree with these remedies, since the medical profession is famed for its reluctance to endorse any healing method until undeniable results and public demand leave no other course open to them.

But I assure you that every case history and every type of nutritional therapy cited in this chapter has been reported by accredited research.

The protein vs. carbohydrate story was merely touched upon in the preceding chapter. Many new facts are coming to light almost every day, revealing the part good nutrition plays in the prevention and control of disease.

Cancer, that enigma of the laboratories, has been linked quite definitely to overconsumption of carbohydrates. However, this does not mean that anyone with cancer can cure his disease by cutting down on the amount of sugars and starches in the diet.

Yet it does mean that possible insurance against developing cancer lies in this dietary credo: "I must eat very little carbohydrate foods; I must be sure to obtain my full bodily needs of protein, minerals and vitamins (especially riboflavin) I must take plenty of light exercise in the open air; I must not overeat at mealtime or by snacking between meals."

These admonitions are based on the knowledge that chronic irritations, and other causes of cancer, have less chance of stirring up riotous malignancies if the body is not overstocked with carbohydrate food substances.

An important, far-reaching experiment has been conducted at the McArdle Memorial Laboratory for Cancer Research, University of

Wisconsin, and at the Michael Reese Hospital in Chicago. A yellow chemical called benzpyrene is known to cause skin cancer in 72 out of 100 well-fed laboratory animals within six months.

There is nothing particularly startling in this phase of the experiment, since benzpyrene is a powerful irritant. But this is the astonishing part of the discovery: If those 100 laboratory animals had been fed 40 percent fewer calories during the time they were exposed to the benzpyrene, only 10 of them instead of 72 would have developed cancer!

The diets given the animals that proved highly resistant to cancer contained a full quota of proteins, minerals, vitamins and fats, but these animals received little more than half as many calories as the animals that did develop cancer.

This reduction in calories was accomplished without taking away the essential food elements; merely subtracting most of the carbohydrates reduced the calories, and yet left the diet fortified with all necessary nutritive substances.

The experiment has been repeated over and over again, and always with the same results: The group of animals receiving fewer carbohydrates developed the fewest number of cancers!

Biologists have good reason to believe that cancer development begins with the formation of a single cell which is abnormal because it lacks normal proteins, or because of a disturbance in hormone balance, plus other reasons not yet explored.

During the so-called "critical" period of cancer development (which immediately precedes the stage at which the disease can be detected by either the patient or the doctor) the cancerous cells must compete with normal body cells for nourishment. If there is only enough food for the normal cells, the cancer cells will be starved out.

This is true because, at the start of the critical period, the cancerous cells have not yet had time to establish their own direct blood supply, as they do during the final or progressive period.

Therefore, since they cannot receive food directly from their own blood supply, the cancerous cells must enter into competition with the healthy cells for the nourishment present in the fluids brought to the tissues by the bloodstream.

At this stage of cancer, the normal cells have a better chance of survival, since they are still the more vigorous cells. The growth requirements for abnormal (cancer) cells are quite different from those of healthy cells.

For this reason, whatever nourishment is present will be taken up at once by the normal body cells, leaving the cancerous cells to thrive as best they can on whatever surplus food there may be. Naturally, if there is no surplus nourishment, the cancerous cells must starve and die.

But, if there is a superabundance of body sugars in the tissue fluids, derived from carbohydrate foods in the diet, then the cancerous cells will have found the nourishment to make them grow and thrive, and the abnormal growth progresses to its third and final stage.

Chapter 2

High Protein Meals

After a high protein meal, with an absolute minimum of carbohydrates, there will be only sufficient food energy in the bloodstream to nourish the healthy cells of the body. When the blood sugars decline to a low level between meals, the cancer cells do not get a chance to live.

That is why overeating at one meal, thereby creating a large reserve of energy sugar, or indulging in between-meal snacks that add all those extra calories, will establish the ideal conditions under which cancerous cells can form and thrive.

When the diet is more than ample in calories, containing a lot of sugars and starches, the cancerous cells no longer need to compete with healthy cells for nourishment.

There is more than enough for everybody, and the abnormal cells come out the winner, gradually killing off the healthy cells by the toxic substances they give off.

That is why those who know will tell you that cancer is more prevalent in temperate climates where the diets are high in carbohydrates.

Among the Navajo and Hopi Indians of our Southwest, only 36 cases of malignant cancer were found among 30,000 patients admitted to hospitals. In the same number of white persons, approximately 1,800 cases of cancer would have been discovered.

This means that the cancer rate among these Indians is startlingly lower than anywhere else in the United States. Why? That is what a group of medical researchers want to find out.

Diet can offer one possible explanation. We know that these Indians do not overeat; in fact, their diet would seem decidedly inadequate to most of us. Also, they are protein eaters, consuming very little carbohydrate.

Moreover, they lead an active, outdoor life that precludes much possibility of their piling up any large reserves of unburned "fuel" in the body with which to nourish and promote the growth of cancerous cells.

It is also interesting to note that among these Navajo and Hopi Indians there is practically no diabetes, and very few cases of de-generative diseases of the heart and blood vessels, such as hardening of the arteries and high blood pressure, all of which can be traced either to emotional disturbances or to overeating.

Another sidelight on cancer has recently been announced by the research laboratories. Riboflavin (vitamin B-2) seems able to prevent formation of some types of cancer.

The connection between this vitamin and cancer inhibition was first suspected when it was discovered that the Bantu black, an African tribe that exists on a diet extremely low in riboflavin, are likely to develop cancer of the liver.

In fact, about half of this tribe dies from cancer of the liver. Continuing the research along this line, it was found that laboratory animals fed large amounts of riboflavin were far less likely to develop liver tumors when given an irritating, cancer producing chemical known as azo dye.

Riboflavin gives a certain protection against cancerous cells, because one of the main functions of this vitamin is to metabolize or burn up, the starches taken into the body.

Therefore, if there is enough riboflavin in the diet, there cannot be piled up large enough food reserves with which to encourage and nourish the formation of cancerous cells.

Since it is impossible to avoid all carbohydrates, if we are to adhere to a diet containing the delicious fruits and vegetables to which we have become accustomed and which, in turn, contribute to our health we must make sure to obtain enough riboflavin in order to "burn" all these carbohydrates before they get a chance to feed abnormal cell growths.

Chapter 3

Protein or Amino Acids

Protein or amino acids as protein is known to the food chemist is coming more and more into its own as a valuable food factor in nutritional therapy.

Experiments using pre-digested proteins (amino acids) have brought effective results in ailments that include asthma, rheumatic fever, rheumatoid arthritis, coronary sclerosis and respiratory infections.

All physical and mental disorders arising from serious protein deficiencies respond favorably to a diet rich in amino acids. Supplementing the diet with amino acids enables the body to replace the natural body proteins which are used up in destroying the toxins given oil by unhealthy tissues.

Influenza, for instance, first causes pain and muscular weakness because the toxins produced by the flu virus attack the muscle cells, and then the toxins go on to attack the rest of the body, causing fever and general debility.

When the temperature rises to fever levels, body protein is destroyed more rapidly than blood sugar, since the amino acids in the cells must be used to fight the poison.

This leaves the patient with a protein deficiency which can be overcome only by increasing greatly his intake of proteins.

Moreover, we know that a high protein reserve in the body, fortified by a daily diet rich in protein, gives certain immunity against disease and degenerative disorders.

Persons who "catch things' easily are low in protein vitality, while those persons who can defy germs as well as mental and physical hardships, and still remain in good health, can attribute this blessing to the good supply of proteins in their diets.

With plenty of usable protein (amino acids) in the body at all times, cell damage can be repaired before the tissues break down and become diseased.

Myasthenia gravis is a serious, disabling disease of the muscles. Persons suffering from this muscular ailment cannot get the voluntary muscles (such as those in the jaw, throat, eyelids) to perform normally because the muscle tissues are exhausted.

In fact, this is often called the "tired muscle" disease. Experiments undertaken at Cornell Medical College and New York Hospital report that victims of this muscular ailment responded quickly to treatment with amino acids.

Explanation for the efficacy of amino acids in this disease is that amino acids increase the body's power to build up acetylcholine, the nerve chemical.

Persons suffering from myasthenia gravis do not produce enough of this nerve chemical to enable their voluntary muscles to function normally.

Therefore, supplementing their diets with amino acids restored the body's ability to produce sufficient acetylcholine to carry the nerve message into the muscle so it could respond to the will of the brain.

We know, too, that high-protein diets are working miracles in curing injuries which, in former years, would have rendered the victim a hopeless cripple.

One such instance is that of an elderly man who fell and broke his back, an injury which not long ago would have meant total disablement, if not death, to a person of advanced years.

However, the physician attending this man was familiar with the value of protein therapy. The patient was put on a high-protein diet, supplemented by amino acids in concentrated form.

Within six months, this elderly man was leading a normal life, completely recovered from his injury; more active, in fact, than he had been for years, thanks to the extra energy bestowed upon him by plenty of protein.

Another remarkable cure with protein, in combination with other vital food elements, is that of a nineteen year old girl in New York who is promised a normal life after facing the hopelessness of a rare ailment called Hans

Christian Schuller disease that literally "melts" the bones.

When the patient was fifteen years old, she experienced a swelling at the base of her skull, accompanied by severe neck pains.

X-rays revealed that sections of her skull had already begun to dissolve. Before long, the disease had attacked the upper vertebrae and the spinal cord was so compressed that the patient was losing the use of her arms.

She was given into the care of a physician who had proved by clinical tests that the difference between the knitting and non-knitting of broken or diseased bones lay in nutritional therapy.

This patient was given hormones to counteract an imbalance in her thyroid, pituitary and sex hormones; mineral supplements were added to her diet to offset a serious calcium deficiency; the necessary vitamins were given to her daily; and her diet emphasized high proteins (amino acids).

Within a few short months, the patient had started on the road to recovery; her vertebrae were straightening, and her dissolving bones had started to heal.

Nutritional therapy had accomplished another common sense recovery.

Chapter 4

Glutamic Acid

Glutamic acid has the power to feed the brain and to keep the liver healthy has extraordinary possibilities in the treatment of nervous disorders and personality problems.

This pre-digested protein offers considerable hope to hundreds of persons who may now be the victims of subnormal brain activity. We know that glutamic acid increases the effects of acetylcholine, the chemical essential to nerve function.

This accounts for the amazing success achieved among epileptic children by treating them with glutamic acid.

The type of epilepsy most responsive to glutamic acid therapy is known as petit mal, which is a slight epileptic seizure characterized by a momentary loss of consciousness, with upward staring eyes and marked twitching of the facial muscles.

Victims of petit mal have a serious deficiency of acetylcholine, that is, their bodies cannot produce enough of this nerve chemical to keep the muscles functioning normally. Large doses of glutamic acid given to these epileptic victims brought astonishingly quick and lasting relief.

Researchers report that administration of glutamic acid to various patients suffering from nerve and mental disorders resulted in increased action of the central nervous system (which includes the brain), relief of fatigue, increased mental alertness and a lowering of the inhibition and fear complex behavior patterns.

Better yet, all these benefits were conferred upon the patients without the corresponding periods of black depression and physical reaction which follow the use of stimulating drugs.

Glutamic acid is a food, a pre-digested protein, not a drug; therefore, its action in overcoming mental and nervous symptoms is not immediate. The inevitably beneficial effects on the central nervous system are brought about by this valuable food element only after long periods of patient, thorough treatment.

This is logical, since we know that the factors which contributed to a gradual slowing down in brain and nerve functions were the result of years of uninterrupted malnutrition.

Food elements build slowly and safely; it is only the drugs that give temporarily quick "miracle" results, paid for by the unpleasant physical and mental aftermaths that inevitably follow the use of any drug.

Glutamic acid is not capable of causing brain cells to increase, but operates by causing inactive cells to wake up and function.

When considering the therapeutic uses of glutamic acid as a nerve medicine, we must also speak of thiamin, the "nerve vitamin." Administration of these two food elements in conjunction with each other brings about better, more lasting results, because glutamic acid complements the vitamin and vice versa.

Victims of mental fatigue, a commonplace malady among those who seek medical aid, will find that glutamic acid and thiamin may offer them a harmless, effective remedy to correct the malnutrition of the central nervous system.

We know that proteins exert a dynamic action in helping burn up unneeded calories, at the same time that they aid in keeping the skin and muscles firm.

For this reason, any sane reducing diet will derive a major portion of its allotted calories from high protein foods such as lean meats, cheese and egg yolks, or from amino acid supplements.

The person who reduces sensibly, not more than a pound or two a week, will have more pep, retain a youthful look because of taut skin and firm muscles, and lessen the danger of damage to the nerves and vital organs, if he or she follows the advice of nutritional authorities who recommend only a high protein diet for melting away the unwanted fat.

Geriatrics is the name of that comparatively new branch of medicine devoted to the health of elderly persons. Geriatricians have found that most persons sixty years old suffer from one to eight diseases, or nutritional deficiencies.

The diets of three out of four such older persons lack even the minimum daily health requirements of protein, minerals (especially calcium, sodium and iron) and vitamins. It has been found by geriatricians that human organs age, not according to the calendar, but according to the diet.

Dr. Crampton, Chairman of the Sub-Committee on Geriatrics of the Medical Society of New York County, says that a "sixty year old man may have a forty year old heart, fifty year old kidneys and an eighty year old liver, and be trying to live a thirty-year-old life."

I do not agree entirely with Dr. Crampton's figures, since the malnutrition which caused an eighty year-old liver in a sixty year old man would more than likely be reflected in a heart and kidneys that also had aged far beyond the man's calendar years, so interrelated is the health of all the vital organs.

The competent physician familiar with geriatrics will aid his elderly patients to overcome chronic ailments and to conserve their health by stressing nutritional therapy.

The patient's general physical resistance, muscular strength and mental alertness may be strengthened by high protein diets fortified by supplemental doses of amino acids; skin and tissues may be refreshed with vitamins; while heart and blood may be nourished by minerals such as calcium, iron, copper and vitamin E, and the blood vessels strengthened through low-cholesterol and high-protein diets.

In fact, geriatricians and those skilled in the nutritional needs of elderly persons say that protein, calcium, iron and thiamin head the list of diet "musts" for anyone over forty.

Chapter 5

Proteins (amino acids)

Proteins (amino acids) restore the tissues of the vital organs, including those of the heart; calcium (in addition to acting upon the heart) keeps bones from becoming brittle; iron assures a goodly supply of rich blood; and thiamin is the age-fighting vitamin of which the nervous system needs increasingly large amounts after the age of forty.

In connection with the mental health of elderly persons, as well as that of all age groups, I want to mention a significant experiment reported from the University of Seville in Spain.

Tests conducted at that institution by Dr. Urra with both animal and human subjects disclose that the midbrain and its neighbor, the masterful pituitary gland, are concerned with the body's use of carbohydrates.

Therefore, consuming a diet continuously overloaded with sugars and starches is bound to overwork this portion of the brain, as well as the pituitary gland, thereby exerting a degenerating influence on the mental and glandular capacities of these parts.

This makes me wonder how much so-called "senility" in our oldsters actually arises in a brain overworked by the traditionally soft, all-starch diet that is given them because a high-protein diet was supposed to be "bad" for those of advanced years.

It is my earnest recommendation that elderly persons be given the proteins which their bodies need in increasing amounts during the years when the natural tendency of the body is to require more repairs than during its youth.

If these oldsters cannot chew or digest high protein foods efficiently, then supplements of amino acids can supply protein in pre-digested form.

The herb fenugreek is another valuable dietary supplement that should not be overlooked when considering the health and nutritional problems of older persons. Apart from its food value, this herb has the therapeutic ability to dissolve stagnant mucus.

In ancient times, the herb fenugreek was both food and medicine to those persons living on the shores of the Mediterranean and in Asia.

The seeds of the fenugreek plant are still used generally in India, while the fresh plant is prepared as greens. Fenugreek was used as a potherb in the days of the old Roman Empire because of its fragrance of vanilla or coumarin.

A test made by Chicago's famous Laboratory of Vitamin Technology revealed that 8 ounces of a tea made from fenugreek seeds contained on an average: 45.2 micrograms of thiamin (vitamin B-i), 74.5 micrograms of riboflavin (vitamin B-2), 410 micrograms of niacin, 266 micrograms of pantothenic acid, in addition to even more substantial amounts of choline.

These vitamins are all members of the famous B-complex group. While the vitamin content revealed by this test could hardly be termed "nutritionally consequential," still it did reveal that a tea made of fenugreek is very definitely a food, especially if used as a pleasant mealtime and between-meal beverage.

Furthermore, Dr. El Shahat of Fuad I University in Cairo, Egypt, has extracted a new vitamin from the oil of fenugreek seeds. This vitamin, according to Dr. El Shahat's clinical tests, has enabled 345 Egyptian mothers to provide more and better milk for their nursing babies.

This new vitamin has been tentatively called "H" for its human lactation-promoting factor. Small doses of this vitamin found in fenugreek seeds increased the mother's milk anywhere from 160 percent to 900 percent over the former quantity.

These large increases occurred during the earlier stages of lactation, soon after the babies' birth. In addition to increasing the quantity, the quality of the mothers' milk was much better, since it contained greater amounts of proteins, fat, sugar, minerals and vitamins, resulting in healthier, better nourished infants.

Before reporting any further nutritional or therapeutic values of the herb fenugreek, I must emphasize that the so-called "healthful values" of fenugreek seeds, as espoused by the drugless school of healing, is open to much controversy from the orthodox school of medicine if, indeed, orthodox medicine cares to comment at all on this herb.

Whenever a "doubtful factor" in the therapeutic field steps into the scene, research must sooner or later prove or disprove any claims held out for a much-heralded remedy.

However, until such research makes more facts available to the public, individuals will continue to conduct their own experiments with a harmless, natural substance, often reporting their results to family physicians who, in turn, can then write papers for the scientific journals.

Dr. Reeder has this to say about fenugreek in his treatise, Medicinal Plants of America: "Internally, it (fenugreek) works as a cooling remedy in fevers. In throat troubles, with great heat in the throat, the tea affords a good gargle.

A teaspoonful or two is sufficient for a middle size cup of tea, which is either drunk or used as a gargle during the day. It is quite harmless and may be used with-out the least fear."

The herbalist writers have long extolled the soothing and healing virtues of fenugreek. I quote from Rosetta E. Clarkson's book Herbs, Their Culture and Uses: "Fenugreek is reputed equal in virtue to quinine for fevers; yields mucilaginous material from soaking in water (which is used) for inflamed stomachs and intestines; it decreases the nauseating and griping effects of purgatives."

The late Dr. Otto Mausert, famous San Francisco herbalist, in his book Herbs for Health lists fenugreek seeds as antichloristic (i.e., an agent for reducing inflammation), as well as mucilaginous.

Both classifications would indicate that a tea made from fenugreek seeds should prove ideal as a soothing beverage in physician-prescribed diets for ulcers, colitis and other intestinal inflammations.

So potent are the volatile oils in the herb fenugreek, and so thorough a job of penetration do they accomplish, that often a decided fragrance of the fenugreek seeds will emanate from the body pores of a person using the herb regularly as a tea.

These oils seek out and penetrate the most remote crevices and creases of the membranous linings of the body cavities where unwanted mucus often collects in excess amounts. The oils are also absorbed into the tissues, while some of them finally find their way into the sweat glands.

Of course, a normal amount of mucus is essential to proper functioning of the mucous membranes that line the body openings and the vital organs.

However, many persons after years of breathing tobacco smoke, dust and soot, and existing on an unwise diet, will often have respiratory tracts and abdominal organs coated with masses of stagnant mucus that gradually become thicker and thicker.

An eye-ear-nose-and-throat specialist in Chicago when questioned by his patients about the reason for the abnormal amount of phlegm and mucus in their nose and throat has one stock answer: "You are suffering from a chronic case of Chicagoitis.

Move out where the coal smoke can't get you, and I'm sure the mucus and phlegm will at least partly clear up."

The best way to describe what happens when the human system becomes clogged with stagnant mucus is to compare it with an automobile engine caked with sludged oil. In cleaning out these hardened accumulations of grease and dirt from the engine, the mechanic will use what is called "flushing oil."

In other words, it takes an oil to dissolve another oil or grease. Similarly, the theory upon which is based the use of the herb fenugreek as a mucus-solvent is that it requires one mucilaginous substance to dissolve another.

However, the action of the herb fenugreek is not that of a laxative or a purgative; it is solely a soothing and dissolving agent.

Special accumulation areas for excess mucus are the tongue, head and throat, stomach, intestines and renal area. The old term "catarrh" becomes, in modern medical jargon, mucus edema.

This mucus edema often afflicts the upper respiratory tract, causing a type of deafness. And "catarrh of the stomach" is actually mucus edema of the gastric pouch.

Apart from its mucus-dissolving properties, I consider fenugreek especially significant from the standpoint of nutritional therapy because it contains substantial amounts of choline. Recent clinical experiments with choline show great promise for this vitamin in alleviating cirrhosis of the liver.

Tests with laboratory animals show that a diet deficient in choline will produce various pathological symptoms, among which are fatty and cirrhotic livers, bone deformities and hemorrhaging kidneys. Rats kept on a diet completely lacking in choline developed nephrosis, that is, serious disorders of the kidneys.

The 15 miles of delicate tubes which make up our kidneys may become congested with mucus. Should that happen, the kidneys which really are less than a filtering plant cannot perform their normal task of eliminating waste liquids.

Pains develop in the back, waste fluids back up into the blood, and the entire body becomes poisoned. Death may result, since uremic poisoning follows a complete breakdown of the kidneys, bringing about stoppage of all body functions.

Associated with the kidneys is the bladder, the urinary "storage tank." Between the kidneys which produce the urine and the bladder which stores it preparatory to elimination, there are two tubes called ureters.

If these tubes become filled with mucus, the urine cannot trickle down from the kidneys into the bladder at a normal rate of speed.

This may cause the victim to have a desire to urinate frequently, although the amount passed is scanty. This need for frequent urination often makes itself felt when one is first in the throes of the common cold.

Because of the irritation caused by the cold virus to the mucous membranes of the head and respiratory tract, more mucus than normal is secreted, gradually working its way through the digestive tract and organs of elimination into the tubes leading to the bladder.

Until this excess mucus is cleared up from the ureters, the victim of a common cold continues to experience the urge for frequent though incomplete urination.

The mucus-dissolving properties of the herb fenugreek, plus its high content of choline, would indicate it as worthwhile for disorders of the renal area.

Another interesting use of the herb fenugreek has been reported to me by persons who claim that after using this herb for a reasonable length of time, they have discovered that their senses of smell and taste have improved greatly.

This is probably accounted for by the fact that the olfactory nerves, where the sense of smell originates, are based in the nose, a region quite likely to be plagued by over secretions of mucus owing to chronic head colds, sinus infections or some allergic sensitivity.

The same holds true for the taste buds located on the tongue, an organ which frequently acquires a thick coating of mucus, thereby shutting off the taste buds from contact with the food taken into the mouth.

When excess mucus in the mouth plugs the salivary glands, they may swell, resulting in a condition that resembles mumps. This swelling shuts off normal secretion of the salivary juices so essential to maximum digestion of carbohydrates.

Often that miserable condition known as "indigestion" can be the result of salivary glands so plugged with accumulations of mucus and backed-up saliva that carbohydrates do not receive that first digestive processing treatment in the mouth while being masticated.

It is a great favor to the digestive organs to keep the salivary glands free from mucus plugs so they may function freely at all times. Incidentally, one sign of improperly functioning salivary glands is the sensation of a dry mouth and throat upon awakening.

Many individual have reported to me that drinking at least one cup of a tea made from fenugreek seeds each day, and especially before retiring at night, relieves the symptoms brought on by underactive salivary glands.

I am often asked "what is the best time of day to drink tea made from the herb fenugreek." There is no "best time," since a beverage made from fenugreek seeds may be taken at any time after meals as a pleasant substitute for tea or coffee, between meals as a relaxing drink at mid-morning or during the afternoon, or as a warm drink before retiring.

The addition of honey and lemon juice to the tea enhances the natural flavor and aroma of the herb, besides adding extra nutritional value.

Which reminds me; I have a letter from a woman suggesting a new use for fenugreek seeds. "After the tea was poured from the fenugreek seeds," she writes, "they reminded me of a breakfast food so much that I could not resist trying it as such, so the following morning I served myself the seeds with cream, honey and sliced peaches.

And it was as good, if not better, than most breakfast foods." I have no doubt that this woman receives far more nutritional value from her breakfast "cereal" of fenugreek seeds than is contained in the starchy, devitalized products so widely popularized as "pep foods."

As my audiences have learned by now, I personally am against cow's milk in the human diet. Without going too much into detail, my aversion to sweet milk is based on the fact that the adult human stomach is not equipped with rennet, as is the calf's stomach, in order to break down the milk into easily digested curds.

After drinking a glass of sweet cow's milk, you may consider your digestion excellent if, at the end of an hour, even one-third of it is digested; and, at the end of three hours, perhaps less than half the milk will be disposed of in the stomach.

However, buttermilk (either churned or artificially soured) is another matter, since the chemical changes have rendered the milk more digestible. The characteristically sour taste of buttermilk, yogurt or acidophilus milk comes from its lactic acid content.

Chapter 6

Lactic Acid with Glutamic Acid

Lactic acid along with glutamic acid, thiamin and glucose is also a food needed by the brain for maximum brain power. Medical scientists at Duke University have verified my theory that lactic acid influences brain and nerve functions and contributes to mental health.

Incidentally, the so-called shock treatments for mental illness do nothing more than to raise the amount of lactic acid in the blood. Therefore, lactic acid tablets or large amounts of buttermilk can accomplish the same results by a far safer, saner method.

Furthermore, the value of walking and mild exercise in the treatment of certain

55

mental and nervous disorders seems to be the increased amount of lactic acid in the blood. And so, for those patients who are prevented from indulging in this form of mild exercise, lactic acid will often accomplish the same benefits.

Lactic acid in tablet form has the advantage of conferring the benefits of sour milk products on those who have a marked aversion to the taste, or who cannot tolerate the quantity of liquid which drinking the original product would necessitate.

Certainly there is far more food and therapeutic value in soured milk than in sweet milk because of its greater digestibility.

Yet a false demand for sweet milk has been created throughout this country in the past several decades, for commercial reasons. The adult consumption of sweet milk is out of all proportion to the nutritional needs of later years.

Only the other day I read where a prominent physician recommended at least a quart of sweet milk a day for elderly persons.

I wonder if this physician took into account the fact that milk, being alkaline, counteracts the acidity of the stomach and certainly the greater number of older persons suffer from far too little acid in the stomach.

Also, I wonder if he considered the difficulty that the aging stomach might have in digesting such a quantity of milk. Many instances of digestive disturbances in the older age group can be traced directly to a too liberal consumption of sweet milk, since the acid gastric juices needed to digest protein have been neutralized by the alkaline milk.

If you must drink milk with your meals, make sure it is either buttermilk, or one of the other sour milk products.

And if you want the benefits of sour milk without its taste or quantity; then lactic acid in concentrated form can be equally as nourishing. The calcium lost by not drinking sweet milk can be replaced by the use of calcium concentrates.

No therapeutic discovery has been so exploited as that of vitamins. Thousands of persons waste their money on certain brands of vitamins solely because of the hocus pocus which surrounds the newspaper and radio advertising of these products.

And thousands more; skeptical of the ballyhoo, refrain from using legitimate vitamin supplements which their bodies so urgently require.

I do not hesitate to declare that most vitamin purchasers are taking their vitamins blindfolded, without full knowledge of what they do and do not need in the way of these valuable food supplements.

The preposterous number of "new" vitamin preparations, trade names, combinations, potencies, prices, promises and so on ad infinitum do nothing more than to confuse a public that wants to know and understand the truth about vitamins in order to be able to benefit from this common sense type of therapy.

Chapter 7

Vitamin A

Vitamin A, unfortunately, has come to be so closely associated with the eyes and the ability to counteract night-blindness that many persons are likely to overlook its other important nutritional functions.

Vitamin A is also necessary for normal vision and helps prevent an eye disease known as xerophthalmia which causes the lining of the eyelids to become dry, leading to inflammation of both the lids and the eyeballs.

The eyelids, of course, are lined with mucous membrane, and wherever this type of skin tissue is mentioned, immediately vitamin

A should come to mind, since it is known as the "membrane conditioner."

A serious deficiency of vitamin A greatly affects the mucous membranes of the nose, throat, mouth, bronchial tubes, lungs, digestive tract, kidneys and sexual organs.

Eventually the mucous membranes of the entire body may lose their ability to produce the normal secretions needed to protect them from irritation.

Vitamin A, in the form of cod liver oil, was given before the advent of the vitamin capsule with its higher potency to lessen the number of colds suffered during a winter.

This type of vitamin therapy, although it was not thought of as such, is perhaps the oldest use of vitamins with the blessing of the medical profession.

Vitamin A in bountiful amounts in the diet, when properly assimilated, helps keep the membranes of the nose and throat strong enough to withstand the continuous onslaught of bacteria and viruses constantly being taken into these parts via the air we breathe.

Anyone who becomes a ready victim to every cold virus or flu germ that comes along would do well to supplement his diet with at least 25,000 units of extra vitamin A each day.

A scientist friend of mine cured his ten year old son of a tendency toward chronic colds and grippe by giving him up to 100,000 units of vitamin A daily in concentrated form.

The boy was starved for vitamin A, perhaps because his body could not make efficient use of this nutritional element from foods in the diet, so the vitamin supplement offset this lack in his system.

Victims of sinus infections are usually helped remarkably by adding large amounts of vitamin A to the daily diet. This is understandable since what strengthens the membranous linings of the sinus passages will also help clear up weakness and infection in this area.

It is interesting to note that most sinus patients also experience eye difficulties, indicating that perhaps the same lack of vitamin A lies at the root of both evils.

Of course, the supplemental doses of vitamin A taken for the sinuses usually also benefit the eyes, relieving them of a tired, dry, itching sensation, and removing the tendency toward "glare-blindness."

The danger of infections and infectious diseases can be lessened in a body well provided with vitamin A. This applies to ailments ranging all the way from boils to scarlet fever.

At the University of Rochester, laboratory animals were put on diets seriously lacking in vitamin A for different lengths of time.

Disease bacteria were then injected into the animals. Severity of the disease and the number of deaths were in direct proportion to the number of days the animals had been kept on a diet low in vitamin A.

At the University of Toronto, laboratory animals were fed on the same diet, except that some of them were given generous portions of vitamin A concentrate. After a certain time, all the animals were injected with typhoid bacteria.

Three-fourths of the animals that did not receive the supplemental doses of vitamin A became violently ill and died, whereas only a very few of those receiving the extra vitamin A even became ill.

Mothers of growing children would do well to keep these two experiments in mind in order to protect against the childhood diseases, formerly thought to be harmless, but now recognized by medical science as laying the groundwork for many of the diseases and disabilities of later life.

Vitamin A plays an important part in nourishing the skin and the hair follicles; it helps protect the nerve coverings from irritation and damage; it aids the secretion of gastric juices, thereby contributing to better digestion of proteins.

Laboratory experiments with animals have revealed that a diet entirely lacking in vitamin A impaired the nerve of hearing (known as the eighth nerve) so severely that deafness followed.

Moreover, this "A" deficient diet also affected the nerves in the ear having to do with the sense of body balance, resulting in a disorder similar to the Meniere's disease experienced by humans.

A high intake of vitamin A is good insurance against kidney stones for those persons susceptible to this painful disorder.

Plenty of this vitamin and a minimum of foods containing oxalic acid such as chocolate, spinach, rhubarb, black tea, coffee, pepper, bread crusts, cranberries, figs, gooseberries and nuts can help prevent initial or recurrent attacks of this excruciatingly painful disorder.

Persons suffering from exophthalmic goiter the so-called "inward" type of goiter characterized by bulging eyes, hand tremors, rapid heart action and constant anxiety or irritability are being treated beneficially with vitamin A.

The usual dose prescribed by physicians averages 100,000 units a day for one week, reduced to 50,000 units daily thereafter for several months.

The good part about this treatment is that it is not drastic, and in many cases it seems to accomplish remarkable improvement. To ease the "nervous heart" symptoms, thiamin (vitamin B-1) is frequently given with this treatment.

An experiment conducted by Dr. Sherman of Columbia University hints at vitamin A as a key food element toward a longer life.

Using white rats, Dr. Sherman gave them four times the normal amount of vitamin A in their daily diets, with the result that these animals exceeded their normal life expectancy by more than 10 percent. They reached maturity sooner and enjoyed a longer prime of life.

If human beings will respond to vitamin A as well as the white rats did, this would mean an increased 10 to 15 years added to our lives at the apex because of a higher level throughout the years. This would mean a longer period of full activity, with lessened years of dependence for older persons.

These are the almost certain signs of a vitamin A deficiency in the human body:

Unusual susceptibility to colds, ear troubles and infections of the respiratory tract; poorly developed bones or teeth; rough, dry and scaly skin with prominent hair follicles (like goose pimples), usually on the thighs, upper back and legs; skin disorders such as acne or psoriasis, with a marked tendency toward pimples and boils; clogged pores of the face, neck and scalp; inability to adjust the eyes rapidly from light to darkness.

Chapter 8

Vitamin B-Complex

This is a vital, ever-increasing group of food elements that might be called the "royal family of vitamins." Its members include vitamins perhaps better known to you by the names of thiamin, riboflavin, niacin, pyridoxine, biotin, choline, pantothenic acid and folic acid.

Then there are also para-amino benzoic acid and inositol, as well as the very new B-12 which holds out great promise for victims of pernicious anemia.

Thiamin

Thiamin is the vitamin we have encountered previously in this book when it was feeding starved nerves to combat chronic fatigue, and acting on the brain tissues to increase brain power.

Thiamin also stimulates appetite, makes possible a more normal muscular activity, aids the body to utilize starches and sugars, improves peristalsis of the stomach and intestines and helps maintain a normal red blood cell count.

Lack of enough thiamin in the diet may promote or aggravate such disorders and diseases as chronic constipation; dizziness; nausea; insomnia, because of nerve starvation; intestinal disorders; vague headache or neuritis like pains; burning feet; underweight or overweight; diabetes; dyspepsia and loss of appetite; subnormal mental and nerve powers; and beriberi, a disease characterized by general weakness and sudden failure of the heart owing to loss of muscular tone.

An advance warning of an urgent need for more thiamin in the diet is felt in hands and feet that "go to sleep" easily.

In older persons, lack of adequate thiamin in the diet seems to affect the heart muscle, often resulting in abnormal dilation of the heart. Supplemental amounts of thiamin may be needed to protect the heart muscle from undue strain.

Furthermore, many of the disorders that seem to afflict the aging brain can doubtless be prevented, if the diet is rich in thiamin, since this vitamin influences nutrition of the entire nervous system. For this reason, thiamin is also called the age-fighting vitamin.

For the past several years, thiamin has been used to treat chronic alcoholism. The alcohol in the system of a heavy drinker reunites with the thiamin in the body, thereby leaching it of this important vitamin.

This ready union of alcohol with free thiamin takes place because the grain from which the alcohol was made lost all its vitamin B-complex factors during the distilling process, and it soaks up thiamin like prune does water.

This stealing of the body's thiamin usually aggravates a condition already serious because of an inadequate diet (heavy consumers of alcohol rarely eat well-balanced meals), and brings the nervous system to a state of complete exhaustion, thereby creating more and more demand for alcohol as a "lift."

Many doctors Alcoholics Anonymous, too, I am told have achieved encouraging results from the use of thiamin to help overcome chronic alcoholism in habitual drunkards.

Particularly do I urge that middle-aged women (either approaching or passing through the menopause) turn to thiamin supplements instead of to alcohol and drug stimulants for relief of their feelings of nervous weariness.

If you do not follow my plea to cut down drastically on your consumption of sugars and starches, then for your health's sake be sure to increase your intake of thiamin, because this vitamin is needed to help the body metabolize carbohydrates.

Too much carbohydrate, coupled with too little thiamin over a long period, sets up ideal conditions for the onset of diabetes as well as cancer, since we know that excess glucose in the blood feeds abnormal cell growths.

Chapter 9

Riboflavin (vitamin B-2)

Riboflavin (vitamin B-2), when seriously lacking in the diet, causes the lips to crack, especially at the corners, and the tongue to become sore and burning. Sometimes the lower lip itches. The skin may also crack at the angles of the nose and ears.

Because riboflavin is concerned directly with the skin, hair and eyes, any noticeable change in these features for the worse should point immediately toward a riboflavin deficiency.

The elbows may become red and wrinkled, and the skin of the entire body coarsens, showing quick tendencies toward rashes and other forms of skin disorders. The hair may become dull and fall out too readily. Unsightly fingernails split and fissured often disappear after the system receives enough riboflavin.

An abnormally oily complexion is often an early sign that more riboflavin is needed in the diet. This type of skin disorder is known as seborrhea and usually affects women more frequently than men, perhaps because it is the ladies who seem to exhibit more riboflavin deficiencies than do the stronger sex.

The type of cataract known as "nutritional" responds unusually well to treatment with riboflavin. Research at the University of Georgia Medical School discloses that riboflavin was extremely beneficial in preventing this type of cataract, or in checking its growth.

Further evidence of the importance of riboflavin for good eye health is offered by the experiences of two Chicago doctors among the people of a town in Central India.

Therefore, anyone whose eye muscles are weak, or who has a tendency toward eye disorders of any type, should include ample quantities of riboflavin in the diet. It is a mistake to associate only vitamin A with eye health, since we know that whereas vitamin A is concerned with the eye itself, riboflavin acts on the muscles and nerves of the eye.

Niacin (nicotinic acid)

Niacin (nicotinic acid) is best known as the "anti-pellagra" vitamin. But niacin is also thought to have some connection with migraine headaches.

Clinical tests conducted in England and at the University of Lisbon in Portugal disclosed that persons suffering from migraine headaches, as well as from high blood pressure brought on by nervousness, were afforded marked relief after being given large doses of niacin.

A niacin deficiency is usually attended by one or more of these symptoms: scarlet-red mucous membranes in the mouth, nose and throat; skin lesions; diarrhea; forgetfulness; general weakness, accompanied by headaches; and pellagra which is indicated in the early stages by debility, spinal pains and digestive upsets, followed by nervous spasms and mental disturbances.

Pyridoxine (vitamin B-6)

Pyridoxine (vitamin B-6) is called the "tonic" member of the B-complex family, since it is believed to influence normal nutrition, and to prevent certain nervous and degenerative diseases. This vitamin also is an aid to more normal pregnancies.

But perhaps the most important of all its functions is the influence it has on proper utilization by the body of the amino acid tyrosine. When pyridoxine is seriously lacking in the body, a poisonous substance (tyramine) is formed which may raise the blood pressure. Certain types of pellagra which do not respond well to niacin have been relieved by pyridoxine.

Two Swedish scientists, Drs. Antopol and Unna, report that waterlogged human tissues, a condition known as "edema," can result from a deficiency of vitamin B-complex, more particularly pyridoxine.

Lack of this vitamin in the diet may also lead to anemia, inflammation of the colon, certain nervous disorders, irritability and insomnia.

Pantothenic acid is best known to the public, perhaps, as the vitamin that "restores color to gray hair."

Although laboratory experiments with animals did achieve this remarkable result, and many persons who did their own experimenting with this vitamin were delighted with the way the gray hairs in their heads seemed gradually to be replaced with natural-colored ones, still sufficient evidence is lacking to say definitely that either pantothenic acid or para-amino benzoic acid will affect the aging of the hair.

However, there is reason to suspect that pantothenic acid has an even more important function. The precious gift of vitality seems to be tied in somehow with this vitamin, if human bodies respond as well to this food element as does the queen bee.

Dr. Gardner, a New Jersey scientist, has discovered that the royal lady of the beehive owes her extraordinary vitality to the food she receives, since the "royal jelly" upon which she feeds is the richest known source of pantothenic acid.

This may explain why the queen bee lives about five years, as compared to only the three months' life span of the average worker bee that cannot feast upon the "royal jelly" which provides the queen with such remarkable vitality.

Therefore, the vigor, robustness and longevity of the peoples in lands where whole grains are used in abundance may be explained in part by the large amounts of pantothenic acid in such a diet.

Biotin is a rare and mysterious substance. As found in human saliva and in tears, biotin is highly antiseptic.

It also acts to prevent certain forms of paralysis. Biotin seems to be the key factor essential to the growth of every living thing from molds to mankind. Experiments have shown that biotin is also helpful in curing malaria.

Anyone eating eggs should receive sufficient biotin in the diet to avoid a deficiency of this vitamin; however, it has been discovered that a substance in egg white interferes with the body's absorption of the biotin found in the egg yolk.

Hence, anyone who cannot reconcile himself to eating only the yolk of the egg may have to depend upon biotin from other sources.

The inability to absorb fat foods such as cream and butter, especially in children, may be caused by a lack of vitamin B-complex in the diet. Whenever the bowel is unable to absorb fats, the remedies which have proved effective are vitamin B-complex taken in conjunction with liver and choline.

The ability to perform strenuous physical work without undue fatigue is another power bestowed by vitamin B-complex. The Journal of Nutrition reports an experiment made by several Boston doctors with 10 men who were put on hard daily labor at the same time they were fed a diet extremely poor in vitamin B-complex.

Five of the men were given supplemental doses of this vitamin, while the other five received what they thought were the same tablets, but which contained no B-complex at all. At the end of the second week, the men who were not receiving the B-complex supplements had lost much of their physical fitness.

They tired easily, and complained of pains in the muscles and joints; their appetite was poor, and they suffered from constipation. But when B-complex was restored to their diet in ample quantities, these fatigue symptoms cleared up entirely.

Truly, vitamin B-complex is the "hub" around which good vitamin nutrition must be built. To neglect any of the members of this powerful vitamin family is to jeopardize the health of both mind and body.

Chapter 10

Vitamin C

Vitamin C earned its niche in the hall of nutritional fame long ago by being recognized as the substance that prevents scurvy, a disease likely to be contracted by sailors, explorers and others cut off from daily supplies of fresh, raw fruits and vegetables.

Explorers who fell ill of scurvy were taken in hand by the native healers and fed the adrenal glands of animals, a rich source of vitamin C. Or sometimes the patients were made to drink a tea brewed from pine needles.

British sailors, still known as "limies," were made to suck on limes or lemons to guard them against the disease which otherwise would disable crews on long voyages.

Of course, no one in those days had ever heard of vitamin C, but they did know that these particular foods had the power to ward off a disease that started with inflamed and bleeding gums, loss of weight, anemia, and pain in the extremities, followed by hemorrhages in the skin and joints and swelling of the limbs. In severe cases the teeth became loose and fell from the gums.

Scurvy, of course, is not confined to sailors and explorers. It may attack anyone child or adult who lives on a diet that does not include liberal amounts of raw fruits, berries and vegetables, especially citrus fruits and tomatoes.

Vitamin C is essential for formation of the intercellular substances in the bones, teeth, cartilage and capillaries.

In other words, it is vitamin C that helps make the "cement" to hold the body cells together. It is also considered an important agent in assisting the cells to "breathe" the oxygen brought to them by the bloodstream.

Ascorbic acid is the chemist's name for vitamin C. A prominent chemist said recently that "this vitamin is shaping up to be one of the most important chemicals with which we have yet come in contact."

There is sufficient evidence to believe that ascorbic acid can be utilized by the body in many ways which are entirely separate from its specific action as a vitamin.

Any condition that causes the body to speed up its rate of living automatically increases the body's need for vitamin C. This is true in such conditions as pregnancy, over activity of the thyroid glands (known as hyperthyroidism), tuberculosis, rheumatic fever, pneumonia, infection of the bones (osteomyelitis) and other diseases that cause high fevers.

When the body is fighting any kind of fever, the amount of vitamin C in the blood falls rapidly, indicating the need for liberal replacements in the diet.

In fact, some physicians have found that vitamin C may be used to counteract the aches and pains that accompany most fevers; also, that this vitamin is useful in eliminating the toxic substances which are the underlying causes of all fevers.

This is the reason why the person who feels he is falling victim to the aches and pains that accompany the feverish common cold is told to drink "plenty of citrus juices."

Let me add, however, that canned citrus juices are usually as low in vitamin C content as to be almost worthless for this purpose. Only the freshly extracted juice of raw, ripe citrus fruit is rich in vitamin C.

Medical research is leaning toward the belief that a serious vitamin C deficiency is one of the main causes for lowered bodily resistance, a state that predisposes the body to infection and disease.

In a recent experiment, it was discovered that children given a daily preventive dose of 60 mg. of vitamin C in concentrated form were absent from school because of illness only half as frequently as children who did not receive the supplemental doses.

A large school for boys in England found that providing the scholars with ample quantities of vitamin C in both food and supplemental form was of great help in preventing the hitherto regular outbreaks of sore throat, earache, pharyngitis, swollen neck glands, pneumonia and acute rheumatism.

Vitamin C has proved powerful against the virus that causes polio and the influenza "A virus." Monkeys given large doses of vitamin C showed a greatly decreased tendency toward paralysis from virus infection.

In recent years, the evidence keeps piling up on the importance of vitamin C in speeding up the healing of wounds.

One scientist has pronounced vitamin C the most important vitamin in the healing process. Most physicians now recognize the value of increasing the intake of vitamin C before all surgical measures, as well as during the healing of any type of wound.

Perhaps most of its value in this connection is due to vitamin C's importance as a detoxifying agent and a tissue mender. Not only does a wound form scar tissue more quickly with vitamin C, but that scar tissue is stronger than ordinarily formed.

Susceptibility to infection and slow healing of any type wound indicate a nutritional deficiency, especially protein and vitamin C.

Medical science is discovering that a relationship exists between a vitamin C deficiency and certain disorders of the gastrointestinal tract, especially ulcers of the stomach. Word comes from the research; laboratories of Europe that vitamin C may play a vital role in both preventing and treating epidemic dysentery.

When massive doses of vitamin C were given victims of typhoid fever, the death rate was reduced sharply below that which could be expected under other circumstances.

Certain persons suffering from anemia do not respond readily to treatment with iron, despite the fact that theirs is a simple iron-deficiency anemia.

Because of vitamin C's influence on cell structure, one scientist has suggested that vitamin C be given along with the iron to those patients whose anemia does not respond to the usual iron therapy.

Good results have been obtained in many cases of anemia with this vitamin C and iron treatment. A person suffering from underactive kidneys, as often occurs in certain forms of heart ailments and other disorders that cause a dropsical condition, have been given large doses of vitamin C because this food element is recognized as a diuretic (increasing the flow of urine).

Moreover, vitamin C is being used to treat hematuria, a kidney disorder that causes red blood cells to appear in the urine.

One of the body toxins against which vitamin C operates is excessive histamine, the troublesome substance that lies at the bottom of most cases of hay fever and asthma. For this reason, vitamin C has been given to prevent or to relieve these allergic disorders.

However, some physicians claim that vitamin C is worthless in the treatment of hay fever and similar allergic disorders. On the other hand, an imposing amount of evidence is presented by the opposite school of thought.

And certainly those who have been freed from the miseries of asthma or the allergic fevers through taking large doses of vitamin C have no doubt about this vitamin's power to act against histamine.

For those who find no relief from vitamin C for their allergic disorders, let me say that this matter of allergies has its emotional side, too, just as dozens of other ailments. An allergy is often not a simple matter of offending substances reaching the bloodstream because of something we either eat or breathe.

Undue excitement or emotional stress can make a person susceptible to an allergy that already exists, yet remains latent until stirred up by the mind. So perhaps the wise course of action for those allergy victims whom vitamin C does not help is to direct treatment against the nervous system to gain better control over unwise thinking and emotional instability.

Also, Dr. Alvarez, a famous gastroenterologist, after years of treating allergy patients, has discovered that a diet consisting of lamb, rice, butter, sugar and canned pears is non-allergic to almost everyone.

If an allergy is caused by food, two or three days on this restricted diet usually will relieve all the allergy symptoms. Then, by adding other items, one at a time, the offending food or foods can usually be detected and subsequently avoided.

At a recent meeting of the American College of Allergists, it was recommended that asthmatic patients should eat more in order to relieve their wheezing and suffering, since these symptoms also can result from being half-starved.

The allergists say that if the asthmatic patient will eat enough of a normal, sensible diet, his symptoms will be relieved, regardless of his food allergies. This latest finding is directly contrary to the advice given by general physicians.

The allergists cite the case of a twenty seven year old woman who had suffered from asthma for seven years. Her case was pronounced "one of the most intractable" the doctors had ever seen. Nearly every night she had to resort to ephedrine inhalations and occasionally to hypodermic injections of this drug.

In conducting their experiment, the allergists put this underweight patient on a diet of 2600 calories, completely disregarding all her food sensitivities.

Within 48 hours she had marked relief from the asthma; within a week she was entirely free from the attacks and had gained four pounds. She reported feeling better than at any time for the previous three years.

The theory behind the diet that disregards allergic sensitivities is that these food intolerances vary greatly from time to time, so that even though a patient may no longer be allergic to a certain food, he will probably go right on avoiding it, to the impoverishment of his diet.

During World War II, vitamin C earned the name of the "commando vitamin" because of its invaluable power to increase physical endurance, lessen fatigue and combat the effects of heat. This, of course, ties in with what we know of ascorbic acid as contributing to bodily resistance.

Vitamin C aids the adrenal glands to produce the hormone known as corticosterone. And when these important glands are deprived of adequate vitamin C, there is an almost total stoppage in the secretion of this hormone, bringing on symptoms that include an unnatural darkening of the skin, serious loss of fluids in the skin and tissues, impaired kidney functions, loss of body salt, muscular weakness and abnormally low blood pressure.

Vitamin C also influences the secretion of another powerful hormone, insulin, the sub-stance produced by the pancreas to control the body's use of carbohydrates.

Research at the School of Tropical Medicine in Calcutta, India, revealed that the flow of insulin from the pancreas is reduced markedly when the diet is lacking in vitamin C.

The body cannot store vitamin C. This important food element must be replaced daily to prevent a serious deficiency of ascorbic acid. Common colds, fatigue, overwork, alcohol, infections all these rob the body of its intake of vitamin C.

Further, contrary to popular belief, all the vitamin C in our food is not fully absorbed and utilized by the body. Regardless of the amount of vitamin C taken into the stomach, from one-third to one-half of it will be excreted.

Obviously, to assure the system of ample vitamin C for accomplishing its multiple duties, larger quantities must be consumed to offset that lost through the body wastes. Moreover, different persons vary considerably in their daily requirements of vitamin C.

Theoretically, the many natural rich sources of vitamin C should provide this entire vitamin that any person living on a balanced diet would require. Unfortunately, however, we must take into consideration that vitamin C is probably the most delicate, the most fugitive, the most volatile of all the vitamin family; it does not last long in food exposed to light, air and heat.

Within 10 to 15 minutes after an orange is cut and exposed to air and light, a large percentage of its vitamin C content is lost. With this in mind, try to calculate if you can how much valuable vitamin C you don't get in pre-squeezed orange juice that is served in the average restaurant and even in the home, when the juice is squeezed some time before being used.

Then there is the serious loss of vitamin C from out fruit and vegetable crops grown in inferior soils, aggravated all the more by the delay that takes place between picking-time and eating-time, which sometimes runs into months.

Because of the paramount role that vitamin C plays in bodily health and nutritional therapy, and because there is no way to insure that natural food will bring a maximum of its vitamin C content to the diet, health authorities are leaning more and more to this belief: that everyone unable to consume freshly raw fruits and vegetables should supplement his diet with vitamin C in concentrated form.

Chapter 11

Vitamin E

Perhaps the most significant discovery about vitamin E is its recent use in treating serious heart disorders. In an earlier book I reported: "During deficiency experiments with animals, it is not uncommon for an animal to die unexpectedly from heart failure. Various explanations have been given, but it is believed that a lack of vitamin E is generally responsible.

This lack of vitamin E may have a bearing on some cases of heart degeneracy in humans." Even while I was writing those words, Drs. Evan and William Shute and Dr.

Vogelsang of Canada were discovering what vitamin E can do for diseased hearts.

But vitamin E, often called the"anti-sterility" vitamin, has other important nutritional and therapeutic uses. This vitamin is of great importance in the diet as a protective agent for vitamins A and D; it protects and extends the action of these and other vitamins in the intestinal tract and in the body's organs.

When the body cannot absorb and make use of its intake of vitamin A, adding vitamin E as a stabilizer often overcomes this defect.

Diseased conditions of the body brought on by an insufficient blood supply such as thrombosis and phlebitis, chronic leg ulcers, Buerger's disease, and even gangrene in its early stages have responded remarkably well to treatment with vitamin E.

A nine-year-old girl, dying of rheumatic fever, was sent to Canada for treatment by the same doctors who have accomplished such extraordinary results with vitamin E in overcoming heart disorders in older persons.

Vitamin E gave this child a new lease on life, enabling her to walk from the hospital into which she had been carried only a few short weeks previously.

Because vitamin E had proved so valuable in treating certain mental and nervous disturbances arising during the menopause, Drs. Michael and A. Ruggles of Providence, R. I., resolved to try this vitamin in treating other mental disorders.

Reporting in the Archives of Neurology and Psychiatry, they revealed that in a group of 35 psychotic patients (24 women and 11 men), 60 percent showed improvement following concentrated doses of vitamin E.

Especially were the results outstanding with patients suffering from anxiety, decreased ability to talk, and depression agitation.

It is encouraging to hope that this method of treating mental illness, plus the use of lactic acid, glutamic acid and thiamin, as reported previously, may supersede the more violently drastic "shock" treatments.

Laboratory animals kept on a diet entirely devoid of vitamin E soon became paralyzed. Examination of these animals under the microscope showed that their muscle fibers were "washed out."

This experiment brought vitamin E to the fore as a "muscle food," and subsequent experiments, plus numerous case histories, have proved that vitamin E exerts great influence toward keeping the muscles healthy.

Also, this vitamin is valuable in treating the fibrositis that occurs in chronic rheumatism or which often accompanies arthritis. Dr. Steinberg gave vitamin E to 145 patients suffering from primary fibrositis; 143 of them were completely relieved in from one to three weeks after starting the treatment.

Other types of muscular disorders also respond well to vitamin E therapy. Patients suffering from certain forms of paralysis have shown a spectacular improvement after being given vitamin E treatments.

Of course the value of vitamin E in helping prevent or overcome sterility is too well known to need much further elaboration here. Also, vitamin E is used in many instances to stop the rhythmic contractions of the uterus that cause miscarriages in pregnant women.

A wonderful thing about vitamin E, unlike most other vitamins, is that it can be stored in the body for long periods; it does not need to be taken every day in supplemental form for ordinary nutrition.

A good balanced diet will provide normal requirements, but, as a preventive measure, a high potency vitamin É concentrate can be taken once a week to counteract any possible deficiency which may have arisen in the diet during that relatively short period.

Yet, in certain instances of heart and muscular disease, or other bodily disturbances, vitamin E is needed every day in large doses, taken under the supervision of a competent physician.

Chapter 12

Vitamin D

Vitamin D, called the "sunshine vitamin," is the only one of the vitamin family which can sometimes prove "too much of a good thing."

Certain fish oils are a rich source of vitamin D, and their use by persons shut away from the sunshine for long periods is highly recommended. However, vitamin D can be manufactured by a substance beneath the skin when the body is exposed to sunlight.

In this connection, it is interesting to note that a certain oily substance present on unwashed skin will produce more vitamin D during the sunbath than if the body is freshly bathed. Therefore, a sunbath before bathing is more beneficial than one taken after coming from the pool or the surf.

One of the main functions of vitamin D is to aid the bloodstream to absorb calcium and phosphorus from the intestinal tract.

That is why bone deficiencies, such as rickets in children, will result when the diet is poor in vitamin D, even though the diet contains ample amounts of these bone-building minerals.

When vitamin D is missing, the calcium and phosphorus are passed on through the body in the faces instead of being assimilated into the bloodstream.

Other functions of vitamin D include an influence on the parathyroid glands which secrete a hormone controlling the level of calcium in the blood; and upon the thyroid gland which secretes a hormone to control the rate at which the cells use their nourishment.

Constipation, "pot belly," muscular fatigue, extreme nervousness, excessive tooth decay and arthritic tendencies are symptoms of not enough vitamin D in the body.

Chapter 13

Vitamin K

Vitamin K is necessary to maintain the blood level of prothrombin, one of the factors essential for forming blood clots. Lack of sufficient vitamin K in the diet causes certain hemorrhagic conditions, since the blood cannot clot normally to prevent undue bleeding.

Chronic nosebleed can be halted in some patients by administering large doses of vitamins K and C. More than half the patients suffering from this disorder of the nasal arteries are found to be seriously lacking in both these vitamins.

When this bleeding malady is not a symptom of some more serious trouble such as cancer, anemia or high blood pressure, it will respond well to massive doses of vitamins C and K.

A new treatment for chilblains has been found in vitamin K, since one cause for this painful ailment is thought to arise from poor clotting ability of the blood.

A thirty seven year-old man who had suffered from this painful, cold-weather ailment "ever since he could remember" was treated with vitamin K. Within one week his dark red, swollen, ulcerated toes and fingers had returned almost to normal.

Chapter 14

Vitamin P

Vitamin P also has to do with the prevention of hemorrhage, but in a different way than vitamin K. If vitamin P is lacking, the walls of the blood vessels become porous, allowing the red blood cells to filter through into the tissues. This vitamin also appears valuable in helping to reduce high blood pressure.

From Britain comes word that vitamin P has been used with satisfactory results in treating cases of ocular (eye) hemorrhage. One patient had extensive hemorrhages in the retina of the eye, as well as in the nose and bladder.

After being given large doses of vitamin P, the bleeding in the nose and bladder ceased, while no new hemorrhages occurred in the retina, and those present became absorbed. Another patient suffered recurrent bleeding after removal of a cataract, and the iris of the eye became muddy.

Treatment with vitamin P stopped the hemorrhaging and caused the iris to clear up and the entire eye to take on a healthy tone. Further, in this one case, it was reported that the patient improved greatly in general appearance and mental agility.

From this, it would seem that vitamin P will prove a valuable nutritional adjunct, along with vitamin A and riboflavin, in treating diseases and disorders of the eyes.

As time goes on, it is reasonable to expect nutritional research to discover and isolate other vitamin substances. Also, new uses for now-known vitamins are coming to light every day.

The best advice I can give you is to weigh well the claims made for all vitamins as natural medicines, and then to adopt whatever common-sense therapy you feel most suited to your individual needs.

Merely because someone else uses certain vitamins is not sufficient reason why you should do likewise. The only criterion, other than the advice or your physician, is a forthright consideration of your own nutritional habits and knowledge of your own tendencies toward certain bodily disorders and diseases.

There is much to gain in health and vigor by adopting nutritional therapy on a common-sense basis.

Some degree of tendency toward infection and disease exists in all human beings, regardless of outward appearances of health. The degree to which this tendency extends depends upon the constant level at which the general health and bodily resistance are maintained.

Therefore, resistance to infection and disease depends mainly upon the health of our trillions of living body cells.

If consistently well-nourished and properly cleansed of their waste matter, these cells protect the mind and body against fatigue, which, in the final analysis, is nothing more than a diseased situation arising from a conglomerate of ill-used body cells.

For this reason I believe that medicine and surgery are only part of the health story, a sort of addenda that enters the volume after the main story is written. Medicine cannot nourish living cells, nor can it rebuild them.

All medicine can do is to dash to the rescue after the cells have been starved, as well as poisoned by their own wastes.

Medicines are nothing more than uncertain emergency measures. But good nutrition is the solid foundation that gives cell structures the strength and invulnerability that lessen their chances of needing these emergency measures.

Even when a bodily crisis arises, it usually stems from that one universal malady malnutrition. Therefore, the logical attack on the one basic disease is through food elements, by augmenting those already in the diet and supplying those that are lacking.

More and more the healing profession is coming to realize that the approach to good health, as well as to restored health, is through nutritional therapy. That is why I call upon you to make food elements your best medicine both preventive and remedial.

Chapter 15

The Mental Side To Great Health!

There's a mental side to good health that can make our later years a blessing instead of a trial. At This point I am going to step out of character as a nutritionist and health counselor to assume the role of family friend. In other words, I am going to talk to you like a "Dutch Uncle."

My long time, nationwide contact with thousands of persons every year during the course of my lecture tours has convinced me that too many people are in love with death I

Dying has become a "bad habit." Although the urge to live remains strong in most animals to the very last, man seems to resign himself at a comparatively young age to the act of his death.

Particularly am I reminded of the man who, shortly after his forty ninth birthday; began speaking of himself as a man "almost sixty."

When anyone remonstrated with him that a good, long eleven years still separated him from the venerable age of sixty, he would reply, "Oh, well, it's all the same. I feel like sixty, and maybe I won't live even that long."

Actually, this man passed away in his seventy-ninth year, but he had been dead mentally for more than thirty years! Throughout three potentially fruitful decades he had allowed his mind and his personal interests to stagnate, waiting for the death that he was so sure would find him before another dawn.

I would like to be able to feel that this man's case is an unusual one. But, truthfully, it is more representative than unique. Too many persons past middle age live from day to day in voluntary companionship with the idea of dying.

105

Mention some plan or some future event to them, and this is the usual response: "Maybe you'll live to see it, but I'll probably be gone long before then."

Knowing a little about the vast power the mind wields over the physical organs, I wonder how many of us actually will our own deaths!

Without qualification or equivocation, I venture to say that if we worked as hard mentally at keeping well and remaining young in thought as we do at harboring the notion of death, the average life span of our older people would be so greatly extended as to cause wild rejoicing among the life insurance companies.

Speaking of life insurance companies, and their vagaries, I know a wonderfully active woman now nearing her seventy fifth birthday who some forty years ago was refused life insurance, because her mother had died at the age of twenty nine during childbirth, and her father at forty five had not survived a ruptured appendix back in the days before surgery was an emergency measure.

The insurance representative told this woman that her chances of living beyond her menopause were so slight that his company could not afford to take the risk.

However, instead of brooding over this gloomy prospect of a foreshortened life, this woman's attitude was, "Fiddlesticks! I'll live until I die, and God, not the insurance company, knows when that will be."

Therefore, I hope no one is gullible enough to brood over the life expectancy tables published from time to time from "figures compiled by the life insurance companies." No earthly mind; not even that of an insurance actuary can foretell the year of your demise.

Barring fatal accidents, you will live as long as you wish, and as long as you maintain the wonderful temple of your body in accordance with the laws of nature.

And even when the body begins to falter a little after years of faithful performance, no law of human anatomy says that the mind must close up shop and retire behind the closed door of senility.

An alert, active mind is possible far beyond the time when the legs begin to totter and the hands to tremble. The body is a temple, true, yet the mind is the priest in that temple.

Even though the foundation of the temple begins to crumble, the priest that is our mind can still exert its powers for the glorification of our remaining years.

But a mind that is in turmoil most assuredly does not glorify a life. This holds true at seventeen, or seventy. Peace of mind has raised the humble to the loftiest heights, and turned sinners into saints; but a futile searching for mental ease has driven the intelligent insane, and blighted the lives of brilliant men.

Up to now, throughout the pages of this book, we have talked about diet and nutrition, meaning food for the physical man.

We have learned that proper nutrition is vital to the health of brain and body. But we also must not overlook the paramount fact that a mind will either flourish or decay, according to our mental diet.

The "thought foods" we supply to our minds are as vitally important to our mental health and, indirectly, to our physical organs as the viands on our plates.

Therefore, we must not neglect the mental side of health. Even more than is true of our physical diets, we are at liberty to choose the thoughts that make up the nourishment for our minds.

Although his captors may force a prisoner to exist on bread and water, they cannot control his mental diet the thoughts that determine whether he survives their cruelty, or goes down under their bestiality in a blackout of insanity.

Only he can decide what kind of thoughts are either refused or absorbed into the innermost center of his consciousness.

For this reason, what you are or are not because of your mental diet is strictly up to you. The blame cannot be pushed onto anyone else's marketing or cooking, since the mental bill of fare we daily set before our minds is the most personal choice we ever are called upon to make. We can dish up dismal stews and worry or we can serve garnished platters of courage and constructive thinking!

Physically, if "we are what we eat," then mentally we live "what we think." Rarely, if ever, does the courageous mind give out the command of "suicide." Nor does the self-pitying mind pause to reason, "There are so many others worse off than I that actually I am blessed in many ways."

If your thoughts are bleak and pessimistic, or if your disposition is emotionally unstable, you can be neither happy nor healthy.

Your soured mind won't let you! And when your mind reaches the point where its chief sustenance consists of surly, cynical, depressed or frightening thoughts, certainly there is no health or happiness for the body and the brain that live under the domination of these unhealthy thought patterns.

In other words, life becomes an endurance contest, until the day when death mercifully blacks out such thinking, releasing an imprisoned soul and quieting a harassed body.

Unless you make up your mind to cultivate positive thoughts and a good disposition, then you might as well face the fact that you are in love with death.

If you were not enamored of the black-robed angel, you would seek and find so much that is desirable and worthwhile in this business of living that you would try to live every day in thought and deed as though it were to be a model day for all the others to follow.

These are not mere Pollyanna phrases that I am giving you. It is sound psychology in plain terms. I could clothe my thoughts in high-sounding professional nomenclature, but my advice would fall short of its goal by reason of its excess bulk.

Because I say to you in simple terms, instead of in complicated language that "you can be what you think" does not mean that there is any less sound psychological basis back of my statement.

There are volumes of case histories to illustrate this truth of life. The men and women whose experiences make up these case histories are living, breathing people like you and the family next door.

What they have done to change the course of their lives by improving their mental diet, you, too, can do because your brain and your body are made of the same stuff as theirs.

A tantrum in a beautiful, young woman may be said to make her "spirited." But displays of uncontrolled temper in an older woman cause her to be labeled as nothing more alluring than "neurotic."

A young man may blow his top and be called merely "hot-tempered," but an older man who indulges in fits of vented ire soon earns the tag of "crabby." Uncontrolled anger in older persons marks them, justly or not, as irascible misfits.

Moreover, what these uncontrolled emotions do to the general health almost precludes the possibility of physical well-being at an age when maximum health of body is the prime requisite for happiness.

Controlling the emotions, or regulating the type of thinking that goes on in the brain, is no more complicated than acquiring any other habit.

When we want to learn how to acquire a habit there is no better teacher than the late William James, American psychologist whose pioneer studies on the workings of the human mind have taught us most of what we know today about psychology.

James says that in acquiring a new habit, or in breaking an old one, there are four important things to do:

- Make the motives for acquiring the habit so worthwhile and so strong that you cannot afford to let your will power break down, since every day that such a breakdown is postponed adds just that much to your chances of success.

- Never allow anything to create an exception in the formation of your new habit, until the habit is firmly rooted in your daily life. The real secret of acquiring a habit is to condition the nervous system by regularity of action; hence one exception breaks the chain of that regularity and means starting all over again.

- Start putting the new habit into practice at the very first moment possible. A habit is not formed by thinking of it; action alone counts.

- Keep alive the ability to form a habit by doing a little something extra each day toward the original habit or an entirely new one. This exercise strengthens the will power and guarantees against a lapse into your former mental inertia.

These rules can well be applied to the habit of controlling the emotions and developing right thinking. I would like to add a fifth rule: Set up a safeguard against domination of the mind by wrong emotions and thoughts; this can be done by having a ready store of thoughts and resolutions to rush in and take over the moment one of the pariah thoughts or villain emotions sneaks in and sets up its tent.

But before you can fill up your mind with thoughts that inspire and emotions that calm, you first must have a mental housecleaning of all the musty, dusty, cobweb thinking that has been cluttering up the attic of your body for all too long.

What are such thoughts? Disappointment, spite, revenge, criticism and condemnation of others, self-censure carried to the extreme, brooding over failure, self-pity, rehashing old troubles, morbid lingering over thoughts of illness or accident. These are negative thoughts that blight the personality and lessen the potential of any life.

This does not mean, however, that such thoughts will not return time and again merely because we will that they stay away.

On the contrary, like weeds in a garden, negative thinking is always ready to crowd in and take over, but these thought patterns

114

cannot become malignant until we invite them to enter, allowing our minds to dwell upon them in neurotic enjoyment.

Too many of our friends have a tendency to introduce negative thinking into the conversations we hold with them; a perusal of the daily paper will yield enough negative thoughts to raise the blood pressure several degrees.

These are things we cannot avoid entirely, unless we are content to shut ourselves away from the world in an ivory tower, but what we can do is to minimize the effect that this type of thinking has upon our minds.

This we can accomplish by deliberately thrusting aside the unpleasant things we hear or read, replacing them at once with voluntarily introduced thoughts of a cheerful, optimistic, constructive nature.

In this connection, I must comment on a tendency that makes persons of many birthdays "old." This is the habit of dwelling in the mournful past. Someone has said that he who cannot let go of the past can never grasp the future.

I do not mean that we should obliterate the past from our thoughts. On the contrary, there is much to be gained by remembering the lessons of the past, as well as its pleasant moments. But memories that burn are certainly not memories that bless.

Now comes the hardest part of this mental housecleaning learning to control undesirable emotions. As we grow older, our emotional habits are pretty deeply grooved into our personalities.

Therefore, it is going to take an earnest job of digging to uproot them from our minds. But the effort will be repaid a thousand times over by the increased health and happiness that will follow a thorough job of renovating your emotional patterns.

The most insidious of all emotions is sorrow. It creeps in quietly, takes up residence unostentatiously, and fastens itself upon the mind permanently. It is all very well to experience a welling up of sorrow because of some personal loss, a grave disaster or a tragedy suffered by a friend.

But the tricky thing about sorrow is that it creeps out of bounds so easily, and before we know it we are feeling sorry for ourselves. The strongest preventive against happiness is self-pity. The art of feeling sorry for oneself has done more to wreck potentially fruitful lives than any other single personality factor.

By all means get rid of that vicious habit of killing your happiness with smothering doses of self-pity. I have travelled far and wide, and have known thousands of persons, both casually and intimately, and never have I found an addict of self-pity who was acquainted with real trouble.

Those whose personal lives were so filled with suffering or tragedy that one felt a sob welling up in the throat at the mere thought of what they must have endured always proved to be the most cheerful, the most considerate, the most hopeful, and the best companions!

Then there is anger, an all-inclusive word that I shall use to embrace the equally undesirable emotions of hatred, vindictiveness, irritability and petulance.

If you were to quaff a slow poison every day, you could do no more to wreck your life, both physically and emotionally, than by indulging in outbursts of anger, or by harboring the by-products of this violent emotion.

In earlier chapters we have seen that anger causes the gall bladder to cease functioning at the time when its bile is needed for good digestion; we discovered that anger is a good promoter of stomach ulcers; we learned that anger causes a cloudiness over the eyeball that can dim the vision; we proved that anger can upset the heart rhythm and increase the blood pressure. Hence, from a wholly physical standpoint, anger is something to avoid like cyanide.

But there is another side to this matter of learning to put a check-rein on your anger. Anger is an emotion that chokes out reason, causing many acts that leave subsequent cause for regret. Anger is also an emotion that dulls the finer sensibilities, resulting in a gross personality devoid of the innate warmth that attracts and holds friends.

I know of no surer way to foster loneliness than by being a "sorehead." If it is your wish to repel people and to live in solitary irritation, then by all means cultivate the habit of "flying off the handle."

Getting older need not mean a curdling of neither the disposition nor a blackening of the outlook on life. "As we get older, we merely grow more like ourselves." Whoever voiced this bit of wisdom certainly tied up the psychology of later life in a few succinct words.

The person who is cheerful and courageous at thirty can also be the mellow, optimistic man or woman of seventy or eighty. Conversely, the individual who is the hothead of twenty-five is more than likely to grow into the irritable pessimist of later years.

Yet the person of unwise emotions is not condemned to permanent habitation with his eruptive disposition he is always at liberty to read the handwriting on the wall.

Deliberately he can set about sloughing off old emotional habits and acquiring a set of safer, saner ones.

Our emotional patterns thought habits, too are not fixed like the color of our eyes. We always have the choice of changing anything in our mental or emotional make-up that does not conform to our ideas of the kind of persons we would like to be.

Right here is a good place to add a timely word of warning. Remember there is no law of human relations which decrees that our relatives or friends must love us simply because we wear the weight of many years upon our shoulders.

They probably will care for us, but nothing can make them respect and love us except our own pleasing ways and friendly personalities. Old age receives no more respect than its personality merits.

It is one of life's greatest tragedies to see an older person, no longer in position to keep replacing alienated friends with newer ones, who grows more lonely and more isolated from human love and companionship merely because of his or her own selfish, irascible, unlovable ways.

However, intelligence, morality, good looks, courage, and patience all these can be slightly colorless personal endowments if un-brightened by a shining sense of humor. Often the moralists, the reformers and the educators defeat their own admirable purposes by failing to include in their program liberal applications of homely humor.

The parent who "kids" his offspring into obedience and uprightness often achieves more lasting results than the one who gets results by sternness alone.

A priest who had dedicated himself to rehabilitating juvenile delinquents frequently remonstrated with the boys for their prolific use of obscenities and profanity. But his words seemed to do little good.

Finally one day, during a round-table discussion with his group, the good man launched into a flow of profanity that would have done credit to a longshoreman. Horrified, the boys looked at each other, then got up and started to leave the room.

"Where are you going?" the priest asked.
"We can't stay here and listen to you talk like that!" they replied indignantly.

The priest burst out laughing and motioned the boys back to their chairs. "What have you got to kick about?" he said with a twinkle in his eye. "That's what I have to listen to from you fellows all the time."

From that hour forward, anyone could have taken his maiden aunt among that group of youngsters from the slums and not have offended her delicate sensibilities. A little common sense and a lot of humor accomplished what pure moralizing could never have done.

I might even go so far as to declare that a healthy sense of humor is the most powerful antidote for "nerves" that can be administered. A middle-aged lecturer whom I met some years ago was developing "nerves" to such an extent that it threatened to cut short his platform activities.

"I'll never get through this season," he moaned. "I get so jumpy out there before all those people that I want to dash off the stage and hide myself. I hate audiences!"

"How long since you've had a good laugh?" I asked him, somewhat irrelevantly. While he fumbled for an answer, it became apparent that this man had never developed the habit of enjoying his audiences. He lectured at them, and not with them.

His program was entirely devoid of humor. He went onto the stage highly keyed up and launched into his subject without giving himself or his audience a chance to relax.

And he maintained this atmosphere of tension for himself and his listeners throughout the entire evening. I am sure that his audiences must have left the lecture hall as nervous as the speaker.

"The next time you lecture," I advised him, "have some fun. Tell a joke or two, preferably one on yourself, and let the audience join in the laugh on you.

Then stop once in a while when you feel yourself getting too tense, and deliberately throw in a few asides to ease the tension for both you and your audience. I guarantee that you will soon find yourself enjoying your work and the good people who come to listen to you."

If I could tell you this man's name, you would recognize him as a speaker greatly in demand today because of his ability to hold an audience by creating a bond of good will between himself and his listeners.

This he accomplishes solely by the habit of sprinkling his subjects with enough humor to leaven the evening with wholesome laughter.

He enjoys his work, and the audiences enjoy him. But this change from his former somber attitude was not easy; he had to acquire a sense of humor.

As this man tells it, he achieved this worthwhile objective by jettisoning a good portion of his sense of self-importance. In other words, when he had learned how to laugh at his own foibles and mistakes, he had laid the groundwork for a healthy sense of humor.

Sometimes the beginning step in developing a sense of humor is merely learning how to smile. Honestly, how long has it been since you smiled because of the joy of living? How long has it been since the antics of a child or a kitten brought a spontaneous smile to your lips? When you catch a glimpse of your face in a mirror, is the expression tense and defiant, or is it relaxed and smiling?

A visit to a home for the aged gave me a valuable lesson in what it means to smile. Among a group of oldsters sitting on a large sun-porch was a woman whose smiling face reached out to me like sunshine in a dark room.

Amid that group of glum countenances, this woman's expression of happiness rose like a pillar of triumph. Unfortunately, I did not have an opportunity to talk with any of the group, but later I commented to the matron in charge, "I must tell you how impressed I was by the expression of good humor and cheerfulness on the face of that little old lady sitting next to the door.

Too bad all older people can't reach a good, ripe age without having any more trouble than apparently has touched this woman."

"You must mean Mrs. Doll," she said. "But whatever gave you the idea that she's never had much trouble? She can neither hear nor speak since a stroke several years ago, and her eyesight is failing rapidly.

Furthermore, since she was sent here nearly two years ago by her son and his wife, not a member of her family has been here once to visit her. She is desperately lonely and afraid of the further isolation that blindness will bring upon her, but not a word of complaint ever passes her lips. She sits and smiles and all of us love her for it."

No matter what your situation or how frustrating the circumstances in which you find yourself, there is always something to smile about, even to laugh at.

A young American aviator named Barry, who was shot down over Germany during the early days of the war and sent to one of the most miserable prisoner-of war camps in that country, tells a joke on himself that has a tear in it.

The food in this camp was not only scanty but barely palatable. At infrequent intervals, the prisoners were allowed to receive a piece of chocolate through the International Red Cross.

But Barry did not eat his chocolate when he received it. Instead, he hoarded it carefully against the day when he planned to eat it all at once in order to gain enough strength to make a break for freedom.

Then one night, when his pile of hoarded chocolate was assuming encouraging proportions, the air raid sirens sounded a warning of allied planes overhead.

Barry's first thought was of his chocolate. He didn't want to die and leave behind all that sweetness untasted! Quickly, he brought the candy forth from its cache and stuffed it into his mouth as fast as he could.

Before the last lingering deliciousness had left his tongue, the all-clear signal sounded; it had been a false alarm. Barry hadn't been in danger of being killed after all, and now his carefully hoarded chocolate was gone.

"Oh, well, I thought to myself," as he now tells it, "maybe the chocolate will do me good anyhow but just then I had to make a dash for outside. Have you ever been seasick on chocolate? I was.

Quite a while later, when I was able to get my stomach back in place, I lay on the ground and howled with laughter at the picture I must have made, standing in the deserted barracks, stuffing chocolate into my face like a kid let loose in a candy store."

Surely a sense of humor saved Barry from some pretty morbid thoughts in surroundings which might well have driven a less balanced mind insane.

This matter of staying young mentally despite the tell-tale calendar is worth striving to achieve. Not only does a youthful mental outlook brighten our latter days, it also acts to multiply those days into a longer life.

I have met and talked with many persons whose years numbered into the nineties, and even some who had passed the century mark. As I look back now on these oldsters, the one trait which all of them seemed to share in common was that of enthusiasm.

One ninety-five-year-old woman had just started a collection of British stamps as a gesture toward the highly enjoyable trip she had made to the British Isles all alone at the age of eighty.

She talked to me as eagerly about her stamp hobby as my own young sons might have. A man who already had lived one hundred and four years was writing his memoirs of local and national events in order to have a basis for comparing the events of the future.

"I might forget the significant historical events I have witnessed and lived through," he said, "so I thought I'd better write them down while I still remember them, and then I'll have something to refer to as new political and social problems arise."

Truly this man possessed a mind as keen as, if not keener than, many had come in contact with during my college days.

A mental diet must include "food" to produce such youthful enthusiasm. I know of no mental provender as stimulating to a youthful outlook as an active hobby, or some special interest.

This is advice that might well be absorbed by men and women in their twenties and thirties, as well as those of middle age and beyond. We start getting old the moment we allow our minds to settle.

The housewife of twenty five or thirty who exists solely within the vacuum of her routine duties is older by far than the ninety five year old woman with her stamp hobby, or the one hundred and four year old man writing his memoirs. Wrinkles on the face are far less a mark of old age than wrinkles in the thinking apparatus.

As a suggested range within which to choose and develop a hobby or a special interest, there are the development of manual skills; extended knowledge into an already familiar field, or pioneering excursions into an unfamiliar field that has always intrigued the imagination; or a stimulated interest in social and welfare problems of others.

I would like to coin a special medal for presentation to the Golden Age Clubs and Hobby Clubs established in Cleveland, Ohio, for men and women with minds that want to stay young despite their aging bodies.

These clubs meet weekly for lectures, music, picnics and other suitable recreation. The Hobby Clubs bring out latent or unsuspected talents whose fulfilment would do credit to far younger men and women.

I wonder if the members of these clubs are considerably younger in mind today than they were before participating in these rejuvenating activities.

If other communities throughout the country would see fit to adopt this wonderful program for the benefit of their older citizens, we could make rapid strides toward banishing those twin bugaboos of old age loneliness and uselessness.

Anyone who has regular social contact with persons his own age, and who has proved to himself that his mind is still capable of learning is bound to shed the weight of his years.

At this point I should explain that "staying young" does not mean trying to duplicate physical feats or endurance of a person many years younger. To expect the body to show no signs of wear after years of hard, constant use is not being reasonable.

True, we can stave off the more serious ravages of old age by living according to the precepts of proper nutrition and good hygiene.

We also can preserve our 1920 model car by good care and proper lubrication to keep it in running order, yet only a simpleton would expect to enter that car in the races at the Indianapolis speedway.

Youth can mean something other than physical appearance and muscular strength.

130

The "youngest" old people are those who spend more time in keeping their minds sensibly active than in trying to preserve a transitory youthfulness.

Oddly enough, these oldsters, who forget about the wrinkles in their faces and concentrate on developing the keenness of their minds, seem to be those who look younger than their years.

The best "fountain of youth" is the ability to forget self in the pursuit of the worthwhile things this world has to offer.

Keeping young is not achieved by trying to strain the body back-wards toward a youth that has been definitely outgrown. The adolescent does not yearn to return to a state of infancy; he recognizes that his age group enjoys advantages impossible during the tenderer years.

And the oldster should realize, too, that his time of life confers blessings of mellowed judgment and wisdom that make the mental floundering of younger years seem ridiculous.

Brain specialists and geriatricians urge those of advancing years to keep the mind active throughout life, even though the heart and other bodily organs may become less sturdy as the days pass by.

Drs. Oskar and Cecile of the Institute for Brain Research at Neustadt, Germany, have discovered that mental stimulation is the only way currently known by which our nerve cells can ward off death for themselves.

Whereas other cells of the body can die and be replaced, our nerve cells are created to last a lifetime; there are no replacements in neurons (nerve cells). They must last as long as we need them.

Reporting in Nature; the British science journal, the Drs. Vogt state: "The degree of (mental) activity has a great effect on the aging of nerve cells. Time and again we have noted how the destruction of nerve cells which normally stimulate other nerve cells leads to the premature aging of the latter.

On the other hand the involution (aging) of nerve tissue is delayed by the normal activity of the nerve cells ... in particularly active individuals the aging of certain ganglion cells is delayed."

These two neurologists have noted remarkable cases where great mental activity can bring about the growth of new nerve tissue in brains which had long seemed to be mature.

From this we learn that the brain, unlike the other organs of the body, does not wear out with use. On the contrary, the more we use our brains, the fewer tendencies they have to grow old prematurely.

The inventors, scientists, artists, musicians and writers who have produced their greatest masterpieces at an age when most men and women are sitting with folded hands waiting for death furnish ample living proof to the laboratory experiments of the Drs. Vogt.

That false axiom "You can't teach an old dog new tricks" has helped settle much older persons in self-chosen ruts than any degree of ill health ever could. Yet modern psychology has proved conclusively that the ability to learn drops very slowly until quite late in life.

"Even in a test of reaction speed," says Dr. L. Jones of the British Association for the Advancement of Science, "The average man of eighty is only 50 percent slower than the average man in his prime, and even the latter is less speedy than some men of eighty."

At a recent conference on old-age problems, Dr. Stieglitz of Washington, D. C., stated that age brings many advantages: judgment usually improves, while there is more skill owing to more practice.

The ability to learn is about the same at eighty as at twelve, and memory is nearly as good. There may be less speed in memorizing, but there is likely to be greater accuracy. In the face of these statements by experts in the functioning of the human brain at any age, who can truthfully say, "I'm too old to learn"?

A recent discovery made by Dr. Hersey of the University of Pennsylvania may offer a logical explanation for many of those days when an inert brain makes you conclude that you are "getting too old to be much good anymore."

Dr. Hersey has proved that all of us, regardless of age, travel in emotional cycles which rise and fall from one extreme to the other about every thirty-four days. This cycle ranges from the emotional highs when we look at the world through "rose-colored glasses" down to the depths when we suffer a "case of the blues."

Moreover, the scientist claims that this cycle is as predictable as the rise and fall of the tides. The cycle varies with different persons, but Dr. Hersey says that once you have determined the length and occurrence of your own emotional cycle you can predict your high and low periods merely by checking with the calendar.

To find out what causes these emotional ups and downs, Dr. Hersey collaborated with Dr. Bennett, eminent endocrinologist (gland specialist) of Philadelphia.

After eighteen months of carefully checking and charting the action of glands, blood, liver and other organs, it was noted that the rises and falls in the emotional chart corresponded with that of the physical mechanism.

Particularly did the lines denoting the emotional variations parallel those representing the workings of the thyroid gland. The activity of this gland and the amount of the hormone thyroxine that is dumped into the bloodstream almost paralleled the fluctuations on the emotional chart.

When approaching a period of emotional heights, thyroid activity was correspondingly high; when entering a period of emotional depression, the thyroid gland had begun tapering off its secretion of thyroxine.

During the war, European scientists worked with medical specialists so that skin grafting and bone surgery could be performed at a period when the patient's emotional rise was high, thereby assuring that he would be better able to stand the shock of these drastic operations.

The reason I mention the existence of this emotional cycle is to prove that there is more than a beautiful thought behind the old saying that "it is always darkest before dawn." Actually, when we are the most depressed, our emotional cycle has already taken an upward turn and brighter days are on the way.

However, I believe that we can keep the low period in these emotional cycles from reaching such depressing depths, if we keep the endocrine glands well-nourished and functioning at a healthy rate.

The minerals and vitamins so urgently needed to assure maximum hormone secretion by all the endocrine glands will also help maintain a more normal production of thyroxine, thereby lessening the depressing curve in this emotional cycle.

Any congenital defects with which a person may be born cannot be blamed on the mind. But from the age of reason onward, we create our own physical destiny mainly through the coloring of our mental activity.

Mental tranquility and sane thinking lie within the powers of every normal, well-nourished brain. We are what we eat and think. Good thought patterns and controlled emotional habits can assure a happier, more useful life, as well as one free from mind-induced ailments and diseases.

Therefore, proper nutrition of brain and body, sensible living, and a satisfying personal philosophy are the staff of health that I offer to those who seek either to regain, or to retain, their mental health and peace of mind.

Chapter 16

Brain Foods That Help You Focus

Healthy Diet Benefits

Lacking crucial nutrients in your diets can lessen it may sound trite but it's true: If your diet lacks essential nutrients, it can decrease your concentrate. Not having the right amount can also affect your ability to stay focus.

Make every effort to eat a balanced diet packed of a wide variety of wholesome and healthy, foods. Insufficient calories can cause hunger pangs however a heavy meal may make you feel lethargic.

Fish is a Powerful Mind Food

Fish is plentiful in omega 3 fatty acids. It's also a very powerful source of protein to boost the mind, crucial for mind function as well as development.

These healthy and balanced fats have astonishing mind power: much higher nutritional omega 3 fatty acids are linked to reduce dementia and stroke risks; slower psychological decline; and might play a necessary part in enhancing memory, especially as we get older. For brain and heart wellness, eat 2 servings of fish once a week.

☐

Caffeine, Fish, Ginseng, Or Berries?

Pay close attention to the conversation pertaining to dietary supplements and foods and you'll think these supplements and food can do anything from improve concentration and focus, enhance brain function, attention span and boost memory.

However do they really work? As we grow older, the body ages along with us whether we like it or not. Nevertheless if you include "bright and colorful" meals as well as drinks to your eating plan you could enhance your opportunities of maintaining a balanced and healthy mind.

☐

How Sugar Can Increase Alertness

Sugar is our brain's ideal energy source; I'm not referring to your daily table sugar, I'm speaking of glucose, which your body absorbs from the carbohydrates and sugars you consume. To boost memory, thinking developments, as well as mental ability.

The proverb goes; a glass of something sweet to drink can contribute to short-term boost to memory, mental ability as well as thinking processes. Take it easy on the sugar so it can boost memory, consume too much, on the other hand, you're your memory can be impaired.

☐

Having Breakfast Every Morning Can Fuel Your Brain

Do you feel sometimes you just want to skip breakfast? Research has found that eating breakfast every morning can increase short-term memory and attention. Pupils who perform significantly better than others are those who eat breakfast.

Some of the main brain fuel food at the top of researchers list includes fruits, dairy and high in fiber whole grains. Try not to over eat these brain fuel food; scientists also found that having too much high in calorie breakfasts can also hamper concentration.

☐

Add Whole Grains and Avocados

The organs in the body depend on blood flow, specifically the brain and heart. To lower the risk of cardiovascular disease and bad cholesterol eat a diet high in fruits as well as whole grains and fruits like avocados.

This enhances blood flow and decreases your risk of plaque and buildup, an artless, tasty way to fire up brain cells. Though avocados have fat, it's good for you, monounsaturated fat that adds to healthy blood flow. Whole grains, like popcorn and whole wheat, also add vitamin E and dietary fiber.☐

Did You Know That Caffeine Can Also Make You More Alert?

Sadly there is no such thing as a magical shot to increase your IQ to make you smarter; however there are some substances, such as caffeine, that can help you to concentrate, energize and assistance you to stay focus.

Caffeine gives you that distinctive awaken buzz; although the results are brief. Caffeine can be found in coffee, chocolate, energy drinks, and some medications. Overdo it on caffeine and it can make you frazzled and prickly: more is often less

☐

Blueberries Are Nutritious

Studies illustrates that diets rich in blueberries greatly enhanced both the learning and muscle function of aging rats, making them mentally equal to younger rats.

Research also illustrates that blueberries may lessen the effects of age-linked illnesses such as dementia or Alzheimer's disease, blueberries may also help shield the brain from the damage caused by free radicals.

☐

A Daily Dose of Chocolate and Nuts

A good source of the antioxidant vitamin E is seeds and nuts, which is linked to less cognitive decay as you age. Another great source that produces powerful antioxidant properties is dark chocolate.

Dark chocolate has natural stimulants such as caffeine, which can increase concentration and focus. You can have up to an ounce a day of dark chocolate and nuts and to deliver all the essential benefits you need without the additional sugar, fat or calories.